Evandro Eloy Marcone Ferreira
Rívea Inês Ferreira

Association between anterior spacing and sucking habits

Evandro Eloy Marcone Ferreira
Rívea Inês Ferreira

Association between anterior spacing and sucking habits

Deciduous Dentition

ScienciaScripts

Imprint

Any brand names and product names mentioned in this book are subject to trademark, brand or patent protection and are trademarks or registered trademarks of their respective holders. The use of brand names, product names, common names, trade names, product descriptions etc. even without a particular marking in this work is in no way to be construed to mean that such names may be regarded as unrestricted in respect of trademark and brand protection legislation and could thus be used by anyone.

Cover image: www.ingimage.com

This book is a translation from the original published under ISBN 978-613-9-62388-4.

Publisher:
Sciencia Scripts
is a trademark of
Dodo Books Indian Ocean Ltd. and OmniScriptum S.R.L publishing group

120 High Road, East Finchley, London, N2 9ED, United Kingdom
Str. Armeneasca 28/1, office 1, Chisinau MD-2012, Republic of Moldova, Europe
Printed at: see last page
ISBN: 978-620-7-72523-6

SUMMARY

DEDICATION

*/ my wife, **Andréia**, for her understanding in times of absence, comfort in times of anguish, for her affection, love and dedication.*

THANKS

*To **God**, for his infinite love and for always lighting my way, lifting me up and filling me with strength for every difficulty I encounter. Thank you for making me feel your presence at every moment of this journey.*

*/ my advisor and teacher, **Rivea Inês Ferreira**, for her teachings, for her brilliant guidance in this work, for her commitment, dedication, patience, availability and for having shown me that to be a true teacher, you have to love your profession.*

*To my wife, **Andréia**, for being such a faithful and patient companion, encouraging me day after day and fighting with me to achieve this goal. This achievement is also yours! I love you!*

*To the coordinator of the master's program in Orthodontics at UNICID, Professor **Flàvio Vellini Ferreira**, for his example of professionalism.*

*To my great teachers, **Ana Carla Nahàs, Daniela Gamba Garib, Flàvio Augusto Cotrim Ferreira, Helio Scavone Jr, Karyna do Valle-Corotti, Paulo Eduardo Carvalho, Rivea Inês Ferreira**, for the valuable knowledge they imparted, for their constant concern for excellence and for their great participation in my training as a teacher, my eternal gratitude.*

*To Professor **Rafael Pimentel Maia** for his great collaboration in the application of the statistical tests in this work.*

*To my dear classmates, **Rita, Camilla, Leni, Sandrine,***

***Ricardo, Patricio, Fàbio; Daniel, Mustafà and Marcus** for the unforgettable moments of conviviality and friendship.*

*To my parents-in-law, **Fernando and Fàtima,** for their kindness and generosity in welcoming me with so much affection.*

*My sisters-in-law **Ana and Manoela** for the affection and joy they gave me.*

*To this wonderful family **Silvio, Aparecida, Aline, Bruna and Amanda** who took me in and gave me so much love and affection, I have no words to say about you, thank you for everything.*

To my parents and siblings, who, despite the distance between us, I know are rooting for me.

*/ UNICID clinic employee, **Arlinda Miron**, for always being helpful and kind.*

*To **everyone** who, in any way, helped and contributed so that this work could be carried out.*

Ferreira, E. E. M. Association between anterior spacing and non-nutritive sucking habits in Japanese-Brazilians and leucoderms, in the deciduous dentition [Master's dissertation]. Sao Paulo: Universidade Cidade de Sao Paulo; 2008.

SUMMARY

The aim of this study was to evaluate the prevalence of anterior interdental spacing characteristics in the deciduous dentition in Japanese-Brazilians and Brazilian leucoderms, as well as to test the association between occlusal variants and non-nutritive sucking habits. Two samples of both sexes, aged between 2 and 6 years, were selected: 405 Japanese-Brazilians from 36 public and private schools in the state of São Paulo and 510 leucoderms from 11 public institutions in the eastern zone of São Paulo - SP. The investigation into non-nutritive sucking habits was carried out using a questionnaire answered by the parents/guardians. Occlusal characteristics were obtained from previously collected clinical records. Variants relating to interdental spacing in the upper and lower arches were classified into four categories: *generalized spacing, primate spaces only, absence of spacing* and *crowding*. The horizontal interincisor gap was also assessed to analyze a possible relationship between increased overjet, a history of non-nutritive sucking habits and anterior spacing in the upper arch. The data was submitted to descriptive and analytical statistical evaluations. Occlusal characteristics were compared according to age group and gender in each ethnic group using the Chi-square test (α = 0.05). Logistic regression analysis was applied to verify the effect of the factors age group, sex and ethnic group on the prevalence of anterior spacing characteristics. In addition, a logistic regression model was fitted to analyze the association between the characteristics *generalized anterior spacing* or *only the presence of primate spaces* in the upper arch, non-nutritive sucking habits and increased overjet. In Japanese-Brazilians, generalized anterior spacing was the most prevalent characteristic in the upper (46.2%) and lower (53.3%) arches. The frequency of primate spaces was higher in the upper arch (28.2% *versus* 15.3%). For the characteristics relating to the absence of spaces (21.7% - 26.4%) and crowding (4% - 4.9%), the variation was relatively small between the percentages in the upper and lower arches. In leucoderms, the frequencies of characteristics relating to the absence of spaces and the presence of primate spaces showed a distribution pattern similar to that observed in Japanese-Brazilians. Generalized spacing was diagnosed in approximately 50% of the upper and lower dental arches. However, the prevalence of crowding was 3 times higher in the lower arch (12.8% *versus* 3.9%). Leucoderms were 2.8 times more likely to develop crowding in the lower arch compared to Japanese-Brazilians (p = 0.000). There was no association between the prevalence of anterior spacing characteristics and a history of non-nutritive sucking habits.

Keywords: Diastema; Sucking Behavior; Primary Dentition.

1 INTRODUCTION

Generalized interdental spacing of the anterior segment is the most common feature of the deciduous dentition (ABU ALHAIJA; QUDEIMAT, 2003; ALEXANDER; PRABHU, 1998; BAUME, 1950; FERREIRA *et al*, 2001; 2005; FOSTER; HAMILTON, 1969; JOSHI; MAKHIJA, 1984; KHARBANDA *et al.*, 1994) and accepted by some researchers as favorable to the alignment of the anterior permanent teeth (ANDERSON, 2007; BAUME, 1950; EL-NOFELY; SADEK; SOLIMAN, 1989; KHARBANDA *et al.*, 1994). Although Delabarre (1819 *apud* BAUME, 1950) initially described anterior spacing in the deciduous dentition, Baume (1950) was one of the first authors to propose a systematic classification of deciduous dental arches. Arches with generalized spaces were called Type I and those without spacing, containing only primate spaces or showing slight crowding, Type II. In terms of prevalence, Type I was found to occur in 70% and 63% of the upper and lower arches, respectively.

On the other hand, the presence of interproximal contacts, or even crowding in the deciduous dentition, is not an indisputable sign for predicting malocclusions due to lack of space in the permanent dentition (BISHARA; JAKOBSEN, 2006; BISHARA; KHADIVI; JAKOBSEN, 1995; ROSSATO; MARTINS, 1993; 1994). Silva-Filho *et al.* (2002) did not consider normality and crowding to be mutually exclusive in the deciduous dentition. However, Thomaz *et al.* (2002) explained that crowding in the deciduous dentition is a problem not only from an orthodontic point of view, but also because it is a factor that predisposes to greater retention of bacterial plaque. Leighton (2007), by mentioning that the crowding of deciduous incisors is very likely to be followed by the crowding of permanent incisors, reinforced the concept of this type of deviation as malocclusion. Furthermore, although growth and development promote dimensional and cephalometric changes between the deciduous and permanent dentition phases, some children may deviate from the normal pattern (ROSSATO; MARTINS, 1994). It follows, therefore, that monitoring children with crowding in the deciduous dentition until the permanent dentition would be a method of preventive orthodontics.

Several studies have been carried out with Brazilian children to determine the prevalence of anterior spacing characteristics in the deciduous dentition (CARVALHO; VALENÇA, 2004; DINELLI; MARTINS; PINTO, 2004; FERREIRA *et al*, 2001; 2005; PACE; CHELLOTI, 1981; ROSSATO; MARTINS, 1993; 1994; SILVA-FILHO *et al.*, 2002; SOVIERO; BASTOS; SOUZA, 1999), however, there is a lack of research on Japanese-Brazilian populations. Several occlusal characteristics of the deciduous dentition, in the horizontal, sagittal and transverse planes, have been evaluated, including their association with non-nutritive sucking habits (ITO, 2006; KATAOKA, 2004; SATO, 2006). However, anterior spacing in particular has not yet been studied in detail in this population. Considering that the racial factor may have an influence on the occlusal pattern, it would be relevant to compare the characteristics of anterior interdental spacing in the deciduous dentition of Japanese-Brazilians and Brazilian leucoderms.

In addition, when it comes to anterior interdental spacing in the deciduous dentition, another variable should be investigated: the recording of sucking habits. A number of national and international scientific studies (ALEXANDER; PRABHU, 1998; FERREIRA *et al.*, 2001; 2005; JOSHI; MAKHIJA, 1984; KABUE; MORACHA; NG'ANG'A, 1995; KHARBANDA *et al*, 1994; PACE; CHELLOTI, 1981; ROSSATO; MARTINS, 1993; 1994; SILVA-FILHO *et al.*, 2002; SOVIERO; BASTOS; SOUZA, 1999) was developed without taking into account the history of non-nutritive sucking habits in the inclusion/exclusion criteria. Given that these habits can alter occlusion in all three spatial pianos, Zadik, Stern and Litner (1977) explicitly stated that the appearance of spaces between deciduous teeth could be due to them. It could also be hypothesized that non-nutritive sucking habits are associated with the dimensional enlargement of pre-existing anterior interproximal spaces. However, a possible association of the above should be experimentally analyzed.

With regard to the characteristics of anterior spacing, a study that addresses the racial factor and the history of non-nutritive sucking habits could make a significant scientific contribution to the study of occlusion in the deciduous dentition. It is interesting to note that the socio-cultural condition of a population sample is related to the acquisition of nutritive and non-nutritive sucking habits (GUIMARAES JR, 2004). Caglar *et al.* (2005), in a multicenter investigation, found that 82% of Brazilian children had a history of pacifier sucking. In contrast, 0% of children in Niigata (Japan) showed this habit. The aim of this study was therefore to assess the prevalence of anterior interdental spacing characteristics in deciduous dentition in Japanese-Brazilians and Brazilian leucoderms, as well as to test the association between the occlusal variables investigated and non-nutritive sucking habits.

2   LITERATURE REVIEW

In 1950, Baume carried out a study to evaluate physiological tooth migration and its significance for occlusal development. To this end, he followed the growth and development of 60 children over a period of 8 years. In order to record changes in the deciduous arches, plaster models of 30 children were taken annually. During the period from 4 to 6 years, the length of the maxillary dental arches remained unchanged in 25 cases and the mandibular arches in 23 cases. In the upper deciduous arches, no change in the intercanine distance was observed in 24 cases. Five cases showed an increase of 0.5 mm. With regard to the upper intermolar distance, this measurement did not change in 25 of the cases. Twenty-one cases (70%) showed interdental spaces in the anterior segment of the upper arch, while 9 cases showed no spaces. In the lower arches, the intercanine distance remained unchanged in 26 cases and the same happened with the intermolar distance in 24 cases. An increase in the intercanine distance was observed in 3 cases and a decrease in one case. Nineteen cases (63%) showed spaces in the anterior segment of the lower arch and 11 cases (37%) did not. It was concluded that: after the complete formation of the deciduous arches, their sagittal and transverse dimensions do not change, with the exception of cases in which they are subjected to environmental influences; the two morphological patterns of the deciduous arch would be: arches with and without spaces; the spaces in the deciduous dentition would not be acquired, but congenital; arches without spaces would be narrower transversely than those with spaces; the spaced arches would often exhibit two distinct spaces: one between the canines and the deciduous lower first molars and the other between the lateral incisors and the deciduous upper canines. These were called primate spaces.

Moorrees and Chadha (1965) evaluated the space available for the incisors during dental development in a study of growth based on physiological age. To this end, they examined plaster models of 184 North American leucoderma individuals between the ages of 3 and 16-18. In this work, children were grouped into similar stages of dental maturation with reference to tooth eruption, rather than chronological age. Each tooth in an individual series of models was classified according to one of six stages: 1) deciduous tooth; 2) extracted tooth; 3) exfoliated tooth; 4) permanent successor erupting; 5) half of the permanent crown erupted and 6) permanent tooth completely erupted. The difference between two consecutive stages in the children's series was also recorded. Statistical analysis of the available space in the anterior segment was carried out twice. First, the development of the dental arches on the right and left sides was assessed separately.

Then, data was obtained taking into account the stage of eruption of each tooth. It was observed that the average spacing and crowding curves of the incisor segments, expressed as positive or negative amounts of available space, respectively, showed a sudden change during exfoliation of the central and lateral incisors, resulting in 1.6 mm of crowding in the lower arch of boys and 1.8 mm of crowding in girls. It was concluded that the level of tooth maturation, i.e. formation and eruption, provides decisive clues for diagnosis and treatment planning, as long as the individual growth period is defined.

With the aim of providing information on occlusal conditions at the end of the complete eruption of deciduous teeth, Foster and Hamilton (1969) carried out a study with 100 British children from 10 children's clinics, aged between two and a half and three years, 56 males and 44 females. Using plaster models, they assessed spacing, molar occlusion, canine relationship, horizontal interincisor gap, vertical interincisor gap, crossbite and midline. They found that most dental arches had some kind of space and 33% had spaces between all the upper and lower incisors. On the other hand, 1% had no spaces at all. The most common spacing locations were mesial to the maxillary deciduous canine (87%) and distal to the mandibular deciduous canine (78%), the so-called primate spaces; but distal to the maxillary deciduous canines (76%) and mesial to the mandibular deciduous canines (65%) were almost as frequent.

van der Linden, in 1974, explained that tooth morphogenesis, occlusion development and craniofacial growth are determined by different mechanisms. However, these aspects are interrelated and interact in various ways. All three aspects are related to the phenomenon of dental crowding. Before tooth eruption, crowding is a physiological phenomenon for the deciduous and permanent dentitions. In the deciduous dentition, the growth of the apical bone bases is generally sufficient to allow the teeth to be aligned from the moment of eruption. In the permanent dentition, there is often a discrepancy between the perimeter available in the arch and the space required for proper alignment of the teeth. Considering that crowding is mainly a problem of the permanent dentition, this author proposed classifying it into: primary, secondary and tertiary. Primary crowding refers to the discrepancy between the size of the dental arches and the dimensions of the teeth, which are mainly genetically determined. Secondary crowding is caused by environmental factors. Tertiary crowding occurs during adolescence and post-adolescence, due to late facial growth.

Ravn (1975), also with the aim of assessing occlusion in the deciduous dentition, used 310 models of children from Copenhagen. The plaster models were obtained during the month in which each child turned three years old. The results showed that the most common area of spacing in the upper arch coincided with the primate spaces, between the lateral incisors and canines, although spacing was almost as frequent between the canines and first molars. Median spacing was not so common, although it did occur in 60% of patients. Similarly, the most frequent space in the mandible corresponded to the primate. Spacing was common between all the lower incisors, although the lowest prevalence was between the central incisors. Almost 4.5% of girls and 2.7% of boys showed contact between all teeth or crowding in the maxilla; 27% of boys and 20.5% of girls showed spacing between all teeth in the maxilla. In the mandible, 4% of boys and 6.3% of girls had contact between the teeth or crowding; 15% of both sexes had spacing between all the teeth. It should be noted that spacing was assessed by inspection and no attempt was made to measure the magnitude of each space.

In order to monitor spacing in the anterior and posterior segments of the deciduous dental arches, Nystrom (1981) evaluated plaster models of 91 Finnish children (46 girls and 45 boys) from 2 to 6.5 years of age. Six of the 91 children had generalized spacing in both dental arches at some point during the deciduous dentition. Completely spaced maxillary and mandibular arches were observed in 24 and 14 children, respectively. Completely spaced arches were diagnosed more frequently in the younger groups. No child had both arches completely closed. Three children had completely closed maxillary arches and six had completely closed mandibular arches at some stage of the deciduous dentition. In the anterior segment, the spacing was more pronounced in the maxilla than in the mandible. Although the individual spaces showed a change in width, the average sum of the anterior spaces was slightly modified. Anterior spacing tended to decrease with age in both the maxilla and mandible. In the maxilla, changes in anterior spacing characteristics and changes in intercanine distance were not associated, while in the mandible, a highly significant association was observed. Interestingly, more children stopped non-nutritive sucking during the study in the group in which anterior-superior spacing decreased than in the group in which spacing increased (12 children out of 43 and 2 children out of 25, respectively). However, the difference was not significant. It was possible to conclude that small changes in spacing occurred during the deciduous dentition period. Spacing tended to decrease between the ages of 3 and 6, with the decrease being more evident in the posterior region than in the anterior segment of the dental arches.

In 1984, Joshi and Makhija carried out a cross-sectional study with the aim of investigating the spacing characteristics of deciduous dental arches that showed normal patterns.

Plaster models of 50 boys and 50 girls aged 3 to 6 years in Gujarat, India, were analyzed. All the children had satisfactory occlusion and none had undergone orthodontic treatment. Measurements on the models were made using a caliper. Two types of arches were observed: (I) with spacing and (II) without spacing (87.5% were type I and 12.5% were type II). Spaced arches occurred more frequently than closed arches or arches without spaces. Bilateral primate spaces were not an isolated feature, but occurred when other spaces were also present. The amount of spacing was greater in boys than in girls.

El-Nofely, Sadek and Soliman (1989) assessed the prevalence of interdental spaces in the deciduous dentition in a sample of Egyptian children. They examined 243 preschoolers, 129 boys and 114 girls, aged between 2.5 and 5.5 years. All were apparently healthy, had clinically acceptable occlusion, no decay lesions and no erupted permanent teeth. Type I arches (without interdental spaces) were more frequent in the mandible than in the maxilla, particularly in girls ($p < 0.01$). Type II arches (with spacing between the incisors, but without primate spaces) were very rare in the maxilla, but not uncommon in the mandible. The prevalence of Type III arches, which presented only primate spaces, varied between 17.8% and 42.1%, and was higher in the maxilla. The frequency of Type IV arches (with primate spaces and generalized interdental spaces) was higher in boys (55.8% in the maxilla and 55.01% in the mandible) than in girls (48.2% in the maxilla and 41.2% in the mandible), with a significant difference for the lower arch ($p < 0.05$). The spacing between anterior teeth was significantly associated with the *mesio-distal diameter of the crowns and the intercanine distance. Wide arches and small teeth were related to the presence of interdental spaces. Crowns were significantly wider and dental arches narrower in children without spaces. It was concluded that anterior spacing was more prevalent in the maxilla* than in the mandible and spaces in the lower arch occurred more frequently in boys.

In 1990, Kerosuo carried out a study with the aim of observing the variation in occlusal characteristics in the deciduous and mixed dentitions in groups of children from Tanzania and Finland, in relation to age, sex and sucking habits. The research was conducted in Dar es Salaam (Tanzania) and Hyvinkaa (Finland). The Tanzanian children (n = 580) were from five nursing schools and were selected to represent the high and low socio-economic stages. Two high and two low socio-economic areas were selected and all the nursing schools were located in these areas. The average age of these children was six years and one month (ranging from 3 to 8 years). African children (melanoderm) comprised 83%, the remainder consisted of children of Asian and Arab origin, 10% and 7% respectively. The Finnish children were randomly selected from all children aged 3 to 7 in the city of

Hyvinkaa. All the Finnish children were of Caucasian origin, a total of 575 were examined. The melanoderm children had a significantly lower rate of crowding compared to the Finnish children. In the melanoderm group, 10%, and in the Asian/Arabic group, 4% of the parents reported that the children had a digital sucking habit. In Finnish children, pacifier sucking was more common (77%) than thumb sucking (6%). Among these children, 10% sucked both digitally and with a pacifier. It was possible to observe that the prevalence of crowding in the anterior region increased with age in Finnish children (3-4 years - 5%; 5-6 years - 16%) and melanoderm children (34 years - 5%; 5-6 years - 9%).

In 1993, Rossato and Martins carried out a longitudinal study to investigate the prevalence of deciduous dental arches with and without anterior spacing, as well as their relationship with the absence, presence and severity of antero-inferior crowding in the permanent dentition. Plaster models of the lower arch of 78 young leucodermatics were examined, 38 males and 40 females, in the deciduous and permanent dentition stages. Only cases without dental agenesis, extensive proximal caries lesions or early loss were included in the sample. The deciduous arches were classified as follows according to the estimated spacing/ crowding, which was done by subtracting the present space (anterior perimeter) from the required space (sum of the individual mid-distal diameters of the incisors and canines): Type I - with positive values of up to 1.5 mm and Type II - with values of less than 1.5 mm. The results showed a high prevalence of deciduous arches with spacing (77%) compared to Type II. When assessing those with Type I arches in the permanent dentition, 50% showed no crowding. However, 10% showed severe crowding. When it came to Type II arches, 78% showed crowding (50% moderate and 28% severe). The authors warned that it was impossible to predict crowding from the characteristics of the deciduous arch.

In 1994, Rossato and Martins evaluated the behavior of some dimensional and cephalometric variables, from deciduous to permanent dentition, especially highlighting the differences between deciduous arch wearers with and without anterior spacing. This study used not only plaster models of the lower dental arch, but also lateral cephalometric radiographs of 78 leucoderma patients. In the permanent dentition, although the group with a Type I arch had a higher average intercanine distance, there was a significant dimensional change in Type II arch wearers, with an increase in this measurement. In addition, individuals with Type II arches showed a greater average increase in the anterior perimeter of the arch and a smaller average difference in the sum of the mesio-distal diameters of the anterior teeth. Based on the measurements of the cephalometric quantities SN.GoGn and SNGn, it was found that Type II arch wearers showed a tendency towards moderately vertical mandibular growth. Type I arch wearers, on the other hand, were horizontal.

In 1995, Bishara, Khadivi and Jakobsen carried out a longitudinal study with the aim of determining changes in the relationship between arch length and tooth size, from complete deciduous dentition (mean age = 4 years) to the time of eruption of the second permanent molars (mean age = 13.3 years). They also assessed whether these relationships in the permanent dentition could be observed in the deciduous dentition. To this end, they analyzed the data of 27 North American girls and 35 North American boys, who had satisfactory occlusion in the deciduous dentition phase, no apparent facial disharmony, no dental agenesis or orthodontic treatment during the study period. The mid-distal diameter of all deciduous teeth and their permanent successors, as well as the various length and width parameters of the dental arch were measured in the deciduous and mixed dentitions. A total of 68 parameters were measured and calculated. Descriptive statistics, including the mean, standard deviation, minimum and maximum values, were presented for the various measurements. *Student*'s t-test was applied to determine how much significant difference was present between the left and right sides. Correlation coefficients (r) were recorded between the deciduous and permanent arches. The results indicated correlations between the various variables in the deciduous and permanent dentitions, but most of these correlations were relatively weak (r < 0.7), with the exception of the incisors in female subjects. In general, the percentage of cases correctly classified by the prediction equations was relatively low. It was possible to conclude that the changes in tooth alignment were primarily the result of a reduction in the space available in the arches. The correlations between the various parameters of the deciduous and permanent arches were of a magnitude that did not allow for high accuracy of the discrepancies in the permanent dentition, based on the dental measurements available in the deciduous dentition.

In order to investigate the prevalence of malocclusions in the deciduous dentition of pre-schoolers in Nairobi - Kenya, Kabue, Moracha and Ng'ang'a (1995) assessed 221 children of African origin, 115 boys and 106 girls, with a mean age of 4.4 years (ranging from 3 to 6 years). One of the predominant characteristics was the presence of interdental spaces. The median space was observed in 30% of the children. In terms of spacing characteristics, the authors found the following frequencies: spacing between the upper incisors (69%), between the lower incisors (62%) and primate spaces (85%).

Otuyemi *et al.* (1997) also investigated occlusal relationships and the presence of spacing or crowding in the deciduous dentition in 525 Nigerian children aged 3 to 4 years, 294 boys and 231 girls. Most of the children had satisfactory sagittal, vertical and transverse occlusal relationships. The most frequent locations of interdental spaces were mesial to the maxillary canines (60.9%) and distal to the mandibular canines (58.8%). In 32% of the sample, generalized anterior spacing was observed in both dental arches (upper and lower). The percentage for the maxilla was 37.7% and for the mandible, 44%. The authors found that 24.4% and 26.3% of the children had interproximal contacts or crowding in the anterior region of the maxilla and mandible, respectively.

In 1998, Alexander and Prabhu studied the facial profile, occlusal relationships and the presence of spacing or crowding in a population of children in southern India. They examined 1026 children aged 3 to 4 years (649 girls and 377 boys) in outpatient clinics and school wards. The convex profile was the most frequent for girls (56%) and boys (62.5%). The straight terminal plane was the most common molar relationship observed in both sexes (68% and 66.5% for girls and boys, respectively). As for the spacing of the two deciduous dental arches, approximately 76% had interdental spaces and 3.1% had arches with no spacing. It was found that 76.2% of the girls had generalized spacing in the upper and lower arches. The percentage for boys was 75.7%. This difference was not statistically significant.

In schools in Petrópolis - RJ, Soviero, Bastos and Souza (1999) carried out a cross-sectional study with 400 children aged between 2 and 6 years old, 207 of whom were female and 193 male. The deciduous dental arches were classified according to Baume (1950). Type I was the most prevalent arch, both upper (93.2%) and lower (90.5%), with Type II being more frequent in females (p < 0.01). The combination of upper and lower Type I arches was the most prevalent in the sample (87.2%). Primates were the most common interdental spaces observed bilaterally in the upper (86.5%) and lower (78.5%) arches. There was a significant decrease in the number of children with interdental spaces as they got older, for both arches, suggesting a tendency for the spaces to close.

Melo, Ono and Takagi, in 2001, carried out a study with the aim of evaluating the indicators of crowding found in the deciduous dentition, which could lead to future manifestations of crowding in the anterior region of the lower arch in the mixed dentition. To this end, they examined plaster models of the dental arches and lateral cephalograms of 23 Japanese children in the deciduous dentition (mean age: 5 years) and mixed dentition (mean age: 9 years), who had not undergone orthodontic treatment. These patients had no missing teeth and caries lesions were limited to the occlusal surfaces. Patients of both sexes were analyzed together. Cases that exceeded 4.0 mm in total space were included in the crowded group and those showing less than 2.0 mm were classified as the normal group. The plaster models were measured at 18 points to assess the size of the teeth and the dimensions of the dental arch, using a digital caliper. *Student*'s t-test was used to calculate the differences between the mean measurements. Discrepancy analysis was then applied to search for dental or craniofacial parameters that would best discriminate between the two aforementioned groups. The size of many teeth in the crowded group was significantly larger than those found in the normal group. Discriminant analysis showed that the mesio-distal size of the deciduous upper canine, the length of the arches and the length of the posterior skull base were effective discriminants in separating the two groups. In summary, the normal group had higher values for the anterior skull base compared to the crowded group, and the reverse occurred for the posterior skull base. The larger size of the deciduous teeth was identified as the main indicator in the development of dental crowding. However, the length of the arches and the dimensions of the skull base, especially the posterior one, in the deciduous dentition, should also be considered as indicators in an attempt to predict dental crowding in the mixed dentition.

In Bogotà - Colombia, Thilander *et al*. (2001) estimated the prevalence of malocclusions in a population of children and adolescents, in terms of different degrees of severity in relation to gender and specific stages of dental development, in order to assess the need for orthodontic treatment. A sample of 4724 children aged 5 to 17 was randomly selected from a population that belonged to the Oral Health Service. Based on the dental stages, the samples were grouped into: deciduous, young mixed, late mixed and permanent. They observed that 88% of the samples had some kind of anomaly, from mild to severe; half of these were reported as occlusal anomalies, a third as space discrepancies and a fifth as dental anomalies. Differences between the sexes were not clearly noted. Crowding in one or more segments was the most frequent of all the anomalies recorded (52.1%), and was common in girls. With regard to the different stages of dental development, crowding gradually increased from the young mixed dentition to the permanent dentition. In most cases, crowding was generalized. In cases of localized crowding, it was observed in the anterior regions, most frequently in the lower arch, or in the posterior segments, associated with mesial migration of the first permanent molars. In the majority of patients, crowding was mild (1-3mm, 35%), while moderate and severe crowding (> 4mm in the anterior region or in the right and left posterior segments) was recorded in 17.1% of the sample. The prevalence of spacing was 25.9%. The median maxillary space (2 mm or more; 7%) is included in this figure. According to these authors, most of the occlusal trends that characterize the permanent dentition were detectable in the early stages of assessment, suggesting that occlusal development is continuous. Consequently, a question arises: When should treatment begin? Early treatment is still controversial in terms of cost-effectiveness and functional and physiological benefits.

Silva-Filho *et al.*, in 2002, studied the tooth-bone relationship (intra-arch) in the normal deciduous dentition, estimating the frequency of arches with interdental spaces, absence of spaces and crowding. To this end, 539 children (294 males and 245 females) aged between 3 and 6 years were assessed in the municipality of Bauru - SP. In the sample studied, the dental arch with spacing prevailed (86.65% for the maxilla and 79.96% for the mandible), followed by the arch without spaces (12.62% and 13.56% for the maxilla and mandible, respectively). 6.68% of the children were crowded, with a prevalence of 0.73% for the upper arch and 6.48% for the lower arch. The frequency of crowding in both arches was 0.56%.

Also in 2002, Thomaz *et al.* investigated the prevalence of the following conditions in the deciduous dentition: protrusion of the upper incisors, *deep* overbite, *premature loss of dental elements and crowding. A total of* 989 children between the ages of 2 and 5, randomly selected from nurseries in the cities of Aracaju - SE, Bayeux - PB, Joao Pessoa - PB and Recife - PE, were *assessed* by visual inspection. It was found that 556 children (56.22%) had some of these alterations and that protrusion was the most prevalent (36.1%), followed by deep overbite (16.7%), crowding (9.9%) and premature loss of deciduous teeth (2.9%). There were no statistically significant differences between the sexes (p > 0.05). The prevalence of protrusion and deep overbite was significantly reduced with advancing age (p < 0.01), while premature loss behaved inversely (p < 0.01), with the majority of these losses occurring due to trauma to the upper incisors. With regard to crowding, no statistical difference was observed between the age groups. However, in terms of geographical distribution, the cities of Recife and Bayeux had the highest rates of crowding (p < 0.05). These results show that there are a high number of children who, while still in the deciduous dentition, have malocclusions or conditions that favor their installation, a fact that indicates the importance of educational and preventive orthodontic measures.

Abu Alhaija and Qudeimat, in 2003, carried out a study with the aim of evaluating the dimensions of dental arches and teeth, occlusal relationships and the presence of spacing in the deciduous dentition in Jordanian children. A total of 1048 children (aged 2.5 to 6 years) were randomly selected from 10 preschools in Irbid, Jordan, and examined for occlusal relationships in the three spatial planes. Study models were obtained from 87 randomly selected children aged 4 to 5 (39 girls and 48 boys). The dimensions of the teeth and the upper and lower arches were measured using a digital caliper. Means and standard deviations for tooth/arch dimensions were calculated for each sex. Generalized spacing in the anterior segment was observed in 61.8% of children in the maxilla and 61.1% in the mandible. Primate spaces were significantly more prevalent in the maxilla than in the mandible (69.6% *versus* 51.2%). In the maxilla, the prevalence of generalized spacing was higher in children aged 2.5 to 4 years (61.4%), compared to the 5 to 6 age group (62.2%). For the mandible, the opposite situation occurred, with respective prevalences of 62.9% and 59.6%. The primate spaces showed behaviors similar to those mentioned above, in the maxilla (68% and 70.8%, from 2.5 to 4 years old and from 5 to 6 years old, respectively) and in the mandible from 2.5 to 4 years old (55.7%), as well as from 5 to 6 years old (47.8%). Furthermore, considering the sum of the mean measurements on the right and left sides, the primate spaces were wider in boys (2.8 mm and 2.31 mm in the upper and lower arches, respectively) than in girls (1.93 mm and 1.47 mm in the upper and lower arches, respectively). Interproximal contact and crowding was recorded in 38.2% for the upper arch and 21.6% for the lower arch. This study also indicated that generalized anterior spacing is a common finding in the deciduous dentition.

In order to assess the prevalence of normal deciduous occlusion, Carvalho and Valença (2004) examined 774 children of both sexes, aged between 2 and 6 years, enrolled in public nurseries in Joâo Pessoa - PB. Of these children, 223 met the inclusion criteria, 55.6% (n = 124) were male and 44.4% (n = 99) were female. The reasons for exclusion were: the presence of anterior open bite, anterior and/or posterior crossbite, clinically visible proximal caries, restorations involving proximal surfaces, absence of deciduous teeth or changes in the number, size, shape and structure of deciduous teeth and eruption deviations. The children included in the study were divided into two groups according to age: 2 to 4 years incomplete (n = 125; 56%) and 4 to 6 years complete (n = 98; 44%). The criteria described by Baume (1950) were used to determine the type of dental arch (Type I or II), the primate space (present or absent) and the terminal relationship of the deciduous second molars (straight plane, step mesial to the mandible or step distal to the mandible). The data was subjected to statistical analysis using the non-parametric Chi-square test (p < 0.05). They found that 65.9% and 64.9% of children in the maxilla and mandible, respectively, had a Type II arch (p > 0.05). In the upper arch, primate spaces were present in 83.9% of children for both hemi-arches and, in the mandible, this characteristic was recorded in 51.6% (p < 0.01). There was a significantly reduced frequency of primate spaces in both hemi-arches for the 4 to 6 year age group (p < 0.05). There were no significant differences for the variables arch type, primate space and terminal relationship of the second molars, when considering gender; as well as for terminal relationship and arch type in comparisons by age group (p > 0.05). It was concluded that the most prevalent arch type was II, with a significant number of children who had no primate space in the lower arch, which indicates a greater likelihood of occlusal disharmonies in the mandible.

In their study, Dinelli, Martins and Pinto (2004) carried out a clinical examination and molding of 235 children aged between 3 and 5 years old, belonging to the pre-schools of the Araraquara City Hall - SP. After an interval of one year, the same children were molded again in order to check whether there had been any changes in the dimensions of the deciduous dental arches. Using a three-dimensional digital device, measurements were taken on the plaster models at the initial (first impression) and final (impression after one year) moments. Measurements were taken of intermolar and intercanine distances, as well as perimeter, arch length and primate spaces. Sexual dimorphism, arch type and the influence of non-nutritive sucking habits were also taken into account. The transverse dimensions increased significantly. The perimeter of the lower arch also showed a significant increase, while the perimeter of the upper arch, length and primate spaces remained constant. The distance between the second upper molars showed sexual dimorphism, with larger dimensions for females. For the measurements of perimeter, length and primate spaces, there were no significant differences in relation to gender. Length did not differ in the Type I and Type II deciduous arches of Baume (1950). On the other hand, the diameter of Type I arches was larger compared to Type II. Finger and pacifier sucking habits did not cause dimensional changes in the deciduous arches during the one-year analysis period.

Also in 2004, Ovsenik, Farcnik and Verdenik carried out a study to assess the reliability of intraoral measurements that compute a malocclusion rate to determine the severity of malocclusion in the mixed dentition. The research was part of a longitudinal study in Slovenia, starting with a sample of 530 children at the age of 3. At 8 years of age (mean = 8.5, standard deviation = 0.2), a total of 101 children (44 boys and 57 girls) were randomly selected for a cross-sectional study. The intra-arch assessment involved the measurement of crowding and rotation of the incisors, as well as the axial inclination of the teeth, by a single examiner. The Kappa statistic (k) was used to analyze the agreement between the individual intraoral measurements and those of the study models. Moderate agreement was found for the crowding of the upper and lower incisors and for the axial inclination of the teeth and rotation of the incisors. Systematic interferences were observed for incisor rotation and crowding in the lower arch, which tended to show lower values on intraoral examination. It was possible to conclude that the degree of malocclusion severity, defined by a total score comprising all the morphological signs assessed, showed almost perfect agreement and very little interference between the intraoral methods and the study models. The diagnosis of malocclusion based on intraoral measurements is a reliable method, as are model records, and is therefore suggested as the method of choice for use in epidemiological studies.

Considering the importance of analyzing the deciduous dentition to guide permanent occlusion and preventive and interceptive orthodontic treatments, Kuswandari and Nishino (2004) collected normative data on the mid-distal diameters of the crowns of deciduous teeth in Javanese Indonesian children. The study included 297 preschoolers, 160 boys and 137 girls, aged 3.25-6.58 years (mean 5.21 ± 0.65), selected from 38 preschools in Yogyakarta, Indonesia. All the children had acceptable occlusion. Plaster models of the upper and lower arches were obtained and the mesio-distal diameter of the dental crowns was measured using a caliper inserted through the buccal side, parallel to the long axis of the tooth, at the points of contact. The results indicated that the magnitude of asymmetry between the right and left sides was greater in the distal teeth of a group (for example, greater in the lateral incisor than in the central incisor), and was *also greater in boys (CV = 5.7%) than in girls (CV = 5.35%). The mid-distal diameters of the dental crowns were consistently larger in boys; however, the stability of these measurements was lower* compared to girls. Significant sexual dimorphism was observed for the maxillary lateral incisor ($p < 0.05$) and first molar ($p < 0.01$), as well as for the canine ($p < 0.01$), first ($p < 0.01$) and second ($p < 0.01$) mandibular molars. Compared to other ethnic populations, Javanese Indonesians resembled Hong Kong Chinese and Australian Aborigines.

Caglar *et al.* (2005) evaluated 47 girls from Brazil, 55 from Japan, 57 from Mexico, 58 from Norway, 54 from Sweden, 59 from Turkey and 55 from the United States, at the age of 3, with the aim of relating the type of breastfeeding, the development of non-nutritive sucking habits and the presence of malocclusions. The results revealed a high prevalence of breastfeeding in all the samples, lasting between 3 and 13 months. The use of a bottle was also common, as almost all the girls used it until the age of 3, with varying daily frequencies. The prevalence of thumb sucking ranged from 2% to 55%, with a reduced frequency in North American girls. On the other hand, the prevalence of pacifier sucking ranged from 0% to 82%, with Japanese girls who did not exhibit this habit standing out. The prevalence of normal occlusion ranged from 38% to 98%, with great differences in the figures for different malocclusions in different countries.

In 2005, Ferreira *et al.* carried out a cross-sectional study with the aim of determining the prevalence of anterior spacing characteristics in the deciduous dentition, associating occlusal variants with age and gender factors. The sample consisted of 388 children of both sexes, aged between 3 and 6 years, regularly enrolled in three pre-schools in Sao Paulo - SP. Interdental spacing in the upper and lower arches was classified into four categories: absent, primate spaces only, generalized and crowding. The presence of generalized spaces was the most prevalent characteristic in the upper and lower arches (60.31% and 58.25%, respectively). The frequency of children with only bilateral primate spaces in the upper arch was higher than in the lower arch (21.91% *versus* 10.82%). The prevalence of arches with absent interdental spaces, but without crowding, was approximately 15% in the sample. Crowding was more frequent in the lower arch than in the upper arch (14.69% *versus* 2.06%). For the lower arch, the prevalence of crowding was significantly higher in children aged 6, compared to those aged 3-4 and 5 ($p < 0.001$). Sexual dimorphism was not demonstrated.

Thomaz and Valença (2005) investigated the prevalence of malocclusions in preschoolers, taking into account the factors associated with these conditions. To this end, they examined 1056 children of both sexes, aged between 3 and 6 years, with complete deciduous dentition, enrolled in pre-schools in the municipal public school system in the city of Sao Luis - MA. A questionnaire was administered to parents/guardians to collect information on the child's general health, dietary habits, deleterious oral habits and socio-economic indicators. The dental occlusion examination consisted of visual inspection under natural lighting, using disposable wooden spatulas and a CPI/WHO millimeter probe. The presence/absence of increased overjet, anterior open bite, crossbite, anterior dental crowding and centric overbite were assessed. The data obtained was submitted to the Chi-square test and univariate logistic regression analysis. A prevalence of 71.4% (n = 754) of malocclusion was found, with the highest rates for increased overjet (27.3%; n = 288), followed by crowding (21.6%; n = 228) and crossbite (20.83%; n = 220). There was a statistically significant association between malocclusion, gender (p = 0.045; OR = 1.319579) and pre-school location (p = 0.000; OR = 0.5978378), and it was more common in female children and those from urban areas. With regard to crowding, they found that children from rural areas were 1.5 times less likely to have this deviation than those from urban areas.

In order to assess variations in dental arch width in relation to sucking habits, Aznar *et al.* (2006) examined preschoolers from three randomly selected institutions in six Municipal Health Districts, one from each socio-economic level (high, medium and low) in Seville, Spain. The sample consisted of 1297 children (719 girls and 578 boys) aged between 3 and 6 years (mean 4.7 ± 0.7 years). Due to the large sample, the dental arches were measured directly using fine-tipped calipers. The measurements taken were: intercanine distance and intermolar distance. The results showed that of the 1297 children examined, 82% (n = 1063) had a history of pacifier sucking or still used it. These children showed significant reductions in intercanine (p = 0.003) and intermolar (p = 0.038) distances. The type of pacifier used by 53% (n = 693) of the sample was the common pacifier and 29% (n = 370) used the orthodontic pacifier. The intercanine distance of the upper arch was smaller (p = 0.003) in children who used common pacifiers. It was possible to conclude that, in the majority of cases, pacifier sucking leads to a narrowing of the upper arch, particularly in the canine region. Digital sucking habits, which lasted for long periods, were associated with an increase in the lower intermolar distance. Mouth breathing was associated with a reduction in the width of both arches, but was more significant for the upper intercanine distance.

Again in 2006, Bishara and Jakobsen analyzed the extent of individual variations in changes in the size of upper and lower teeth in relation to arch length (TSALR - *tooth-size/arch-length relationship*), between the stage of complete deciduous dentition (mean age = 4 years) and the time of eruption of the second permanent molars (mean age = 13.3 years). To this end, they examined data from 32 boys and 27 girls participating in the Longitudinal Growth Study in Iowa, USA. The following parameters were measured: the length of the upper and lower arches, on the right and left sides; the mesio-distal sizes of the upper and lower deciduous teeth, as well as those of their successor teeth. Of the total of 59 individuals observed on a longitudinal basis, 29 (49%) maintained their tooth size/arch length relationships in both dentitions, while 30 (51%) changed to either a more favorable or less favorable relationship in the permanent dentition. These results confirmed and explained previous findings that indicated the presence of correlations between the mesio-distal size of deciduous teeth and their permanent successors, as well as the available arch space, in both dentitions. However, these correlations are relatively low and not clinically useful for predicting values. The clinician would then be unable to determine the presence or absence of future crowding from the information available in the deciduous dentition. In the event of crowding in the deciduous dentition, the intervention should be extended until the mixed dentition, for example, after the eruption of the permanent incisors.

In order to analyze the relationship between tooth shape and crowding in the permanent dentition, Imai *et al.* (2006) evaluated plaster models of 40 Japanese patients at 2-month intervals over a period of approximately 18 years, starting at 3 years of age. The results showed that the mean mesio-distal widths of the central and lateral incisors were significantly greater in the group with crowding ($p < 0.01$) and the mean difference was 0.28 mm for the central incisor and 0.31 mm for the lateral incisor. The Vestibulo-lingual measurement of the central incisor was significantly higher in the crowded group ($p < 0.05$). Although there was no significant difference, the lateral incisor was larger in the crowded group. The mean difference was 0.28 mm for the central incisor and 0.20 mm for the lateral incisor. The increase in intercanine distance was greater in the crowded group, although this was not significant. The average difference was 0.63 mm. The authors suggested that there is no clear relationship between the shape and arrangement of the lower incisors.

With the aim of comparing anteroposterior occlusal characteristics and interdental spacing in the deciduous dentition, Onyeaso (2006) assessed 269 children aged 3.5 years - 125 (46.5%) males and 144 (53.5%) females, from the 3 largest ethnic groups in Nigeria (Yoruba, Ibo and Hausa). Eight randomly selected pre-schools were visited in Ibadan and the Lake District of Nigeria. The Foster and Hamilton (1969) criteria were used for occlusal assessment, which included molar and canine relationships as well as spacing. The results showed that interincisor spacing was more frequent among Ibo children (48.4%) and less diagnosed in the Hausa (19.8%). The differences observed in spacing between the ethnic groups were statistically significant ($p < 0.001$). The distribution of *bilateral primate spaces according to ethnic group showed significant differences for the lower arch, being more prevalent in the Ibo (49.4%) than in the Hausa (21.3%) and Yoruba (29.3%), p < 0.001. The absence of spaces in the dental arches was more frequent in the Yoruba group (42.1%) than in the Ibo (21.1%) and* Hausa (36.8%) *groups.* It was possible to conclude that, although no ethnic differences were evidenced for molar ratios, highly significant differences were revealed for spacing characteristics. Interdental spaces were more prevalent in Ibo children.

In 2007, Anderson carried out a study to determine the dimensions of the dental arch (width, length, perimeter and amount of interdental space) in African-American children in the deciduous dentition. It also compared the arch dimensions established for these children in relation to American children of European descent. To this end, plaster models of 217 African-American children (110 boys and 107 girls) were examined. The parameters were measured and compared with historical standard values of American children of European descent. In African-American children, the total amount of interdental spaces in boys and girls was approximately equal, but differences between the sexes were observed in the space distribution model. Girls showed significantly higher amounts of space between deciduous maxillary central incisors (p = 0.017). Boys showed significantly higher frequencies of space mesial (p = 0.041) and distal (p = 0.006) to the maxillary canines, as well as distal to the mandibular canines (p = 0.001). The majority of both sexes (99.1% of boys and 96.3% of girls) presented a primate space, located mesially to the canine in the maxilla and distally to the canine in the mandible. Boys presented significantly larger primate spaces than girls in both dental arches. The absence of interdental spaces was observed in 3.7% of girls and 0.9% of boys, almost exclusively in the lower arch. Dental crowding was observed in only two of the 217 children (0.9%), in the lower arch. The total amount of interdental spacing was approximately equal in African-American boys and girls, but there was significant localized sexual dimorphism. Boys had larger primate spaces and girls had larger upper median spaces. The dental arch dimensions surveyed were significantly larger in African-Americans than in American children of European descent.

3   PROPOSAL

Based on the literature review, there is a scarcity of studies evaluating the characteristics of anterior interdental spacing in the deciduous dentition in Japanese-Brazilians. Furthermore, although a possible cause-effect relationship between non-nutritive sucking habits and increased interdental spaces in the anterior region has been suggested, few studies have tested the association between these two factors. This study therefore aimed to:

- To evaluate the prevalence of anterior interdental spacing characteristics in the deciduous dentition in Japanese-Brazilians and Brazilian leucoderms;

- To analyze the association between the occlusal characteristics studied and non-nutritive sucking habits.

4 MATERIAL AND METHODS

This non-controlled cross-sectional epidemiological study was carried out in accordance with the rules and precepts adopted by the Research Ethics Committee of the Universidade Cidade de São Paulo - UNICID, and was approved under protocol no. 13259823, on May 23, 2007 (ANNEX).

3.1 Selection of pre-existing samples

This scientific investigation was carried out by analyzing data previously collected in other studies carried out by the Orthodontics Department team at Universidade Cidade de São Paulo - UNICID, which have already been approved by the Research Ethics Committee. The information on the samples of Japanese-Brazilians and Brazilian leucodermas was obtained from clinical records and epidemiological questionnaires that are part of the collection of the Master's Program in Orthodontics at Universidade Cidade de Sâo Paulo - UNICID. However, it should be noted that although the information researched has been collected previously, it has not yet been evaluated with the proposed approach.

3.1.1 Japanese-Brazilians

The sample of Japanese-Brazilians comprised a total of 405 children of both sexes (203 females and 202 males), aged between 2 and 6 years, who were healthy and regularly enrolled in 36 public and private nursery schools in various cities in the state of São Paulo - Arujà, Bastos, Botucatu, Campinas, Ibiûna, Marilia, Mogi das Cruzes, São Paulo and Suzano.

It should be noted that this sample was evaluated in two previous studies (ITO, 2006; SATO, 2006).

Children were considered to be Japanese-Brazilians if they were born in Brazil and had at least 50% direct Japanese ancestry, i.e. they had to have at least one parent, two grandparents or four great-grandparents, maternal or paternal, born in Japan. In order to verify the children's ancestry, the above-mentioned studies carried out a genealogical survey, checking the nationalities of their parents, grandparents and great-grandparents.

The total sample of Japanese-Brazilians is relatively equal in terms of gender. However, based on the distribution of the sample by chronological age (Table 4.1), there were higher frequencies of boys at most ages, with the exception of 5 years. In addition, there were very low frequencies of children at the extreme ages of 2 (n = 38) and 6 (n = 31).

Table 4.1 - Distribution of the sample of Japanese-Brazilians according to chronological age and gender.

	Age									
Sex	2 years		3 years		4 years		5 years		6 years	
	n	%	n	%	n	%	n	%	n	%
Male	21	55,3	49	50,5	69	56,6	47	40,2	16	51,6
Female	17	44,7	48	49,5	53	43,4	70	59,8	15	48,4
Total	38	100,0	97	100,0	122	100,0	117	100,0	31	100,0

Considering the low frequency of children aged 2 and 6, the sample of Japanese-Brazilians was subdivided into two age groups: 2-4 years (n = 257) and 5-6 years (n = 148). This subdivision also allowed for a comparative analysis of the prevalence of the occlusal characteristics assessed in two periods of the deciduous dentition.

3.1.2 Leucodermas

The sample of 510 presumably healthy Brazilian children of both sexes (265 females and 245 males), aged between 2 and 6 years, was selected from a total of 1,377 children from six Municipal Schools of Early Childhood Education (EMEI) and five nursery schools located in the east of the city of Sao Paulo - SP (ROMERO, 2007). The participating nursery schools were selected at random, and the east side of the city of Sao Paulo was the preferred area due to its proximity to the Universidade Cidade de Sao Paulo - UNICID and the workplace of the researchers who carried out the clinical examinations.

Of the 1,377 children, there were two main ethnic groups: whites (44.6%) and browns (48.9%). This finding with regard to brown children indicates racial miscegenation. Given that one of the aims of this study was to assess the differences between ethnic groups in terms of the occlusal characteristics studied, it was important to choose an ethnic group with a significant number of participants, or as close as possible to that of Japanese-Brazilians, and which had less miscegenation. The racial classification of leukoderma was determined based on the observation of skin color (white). This classification was also used by Ferreira (2005), Ito (2006), Sato (2006) and Romero (2007).

The total sample of Brazilian leukoderma patients has a higher percentage of girls (52%). Table 4.2 shows that this sample is quite heterogeneous in terms of gender at different chronological ages. There is an absence of boys at the age of 2 and a predominance of boys at the age of 3

(56.1%) and 6 years (56.4%). For the reasons mentioned in section 4.1.1, the leucoderm sample was also subdivided into two age groups: 2-4 years (n = 240) and 56 years (n = 270).

Table 4.2 - Distribution of the leucoderm sample according to chronological age and sex.

Sex	Age									
	2 years		3 years		4 years		5 years		6 years	
	n	%	n	%	n	%	n	%	n	%
Male	0	0	32	56,1	84	46,9	85	44,3	44	56,4
Female	4	100,0	25	43,9	95	53,1	107	55,7	34	43,6
Total	4	100,0	57	100,0	179	100,0	192	100,0	78	100,0

3.2 Research into non-nutritive sucking habits

Information about the children's general health and the history of non-nutritive sucking habits, specifically pacifier use and digital sucking, was investigated in the questionnaires answered by the parents/guardians, according to the model in APPENDIX A.

3.3 Evaluation of occlusal characteristics

In the Japanese-Brazilian sample, the clinical examinations were carried out by two dental surgeons. The leucoderma children were selected from a sample evaluated by three other dental surgeons. It is important to note that the five professionals involved in these epidemiological studies were properly calibrated.

Prior to the start of the clinical examination phase, training was provided for the calibration of the examiners. Calibration included examining the occlusion of 24 children twice, with an interval of 15 days between assessments. This procedure was carried out with preschoolers from one of the EMEIs studied, in a school environment, to simulate the epidemiological survey. The purpose of the calibration was to clarify the main doubts regarding the clinical data analyzed and to standardize the method for evaluating and recording the information on each individual. The data obtained from the calibration were subjected to two statistical treatments to analyze the reproducibility of the tests. The degree of intra-examiner agreement was analyzed using the Kappa statistic. In addition, Spearman's correlation tests were applied to assess the consistency of the diagnoses made by the five examiners, analyzed two by two during the clinical examinations.

The Kappa indicator (κ) tells you the proportion of agreement beyond that expected by chance and ranges from -1 to 1. Minus 1 means complete disagreement and 1, exact agreement in the interpretations. Zero indicates the same as random readings. In summary, the κ index scales estimate that values below 0.41 indicate weak agreement. Between 0.41 and 0.60, agreement is fair, and between 0.61 and 0.80, it is good. Above

0.81, agreement is excellent. It is worth noting that a low frequency of the characteristics studied and difficulty in diagnosis are associated with low levels of reproducibility, i.e. κ indices equal to or less than 0.40.

From the intra-examiner analysis, κ indices of 0.76 to 1.00 were calculated for the five dentists when evaluating all the occlusal characteristics under study, indicating good to excellent agreement between the data observed in the first and second stages of clinical examinations.

Spearman's tests provide correlation coefficients (Rs) that vary between -1 and 1. Correlations are positive if the variables progress together and negative when one variable progresses and the other regresses. Correlations close to 1 or -1 appear when the relationship between the variables is practically linear. Coefficients close to zero indicate a weak correlation between the variables. Coefficients that are statistically acceptable as strongly positive are greater than or equal to 0.70. Rs coefficients higher than 0.90 were obtained for each pair of examiners, considering all the occlusal characteristics evaluated, which indicates homogeneity in the diagnoses made.

The children were examined in their own school environment, sitting comfortably and facing an artificial light source. During the visual inspection of the dental arches, the examiners used disposable wooden spatulas to remove the soft tissues of the mouth and asked the children to perform maximum habitual intercuspation (MIH) and maximum opening. The occlusal characteristics were recorded on clinical forms (APPENDIX B). The upper and lower dental arches were classified separately into four categories, according to the characteristics of interdental spacing in the anterior segment (FERREIRA *et al.*, 2005):

- **Generalized spacing**: the teeth in the anterior segment had generalized interdental spaces, including primate spaces, bilaterally. In case of doubt, the examiner considered that the upper and lower arches should have at least 4 and 6 spaces, respectively, to be classified in this category.

- **Primate spaces only**: these arches had visibly perceptible and bilateral spaces between the lateral incisors and upper deciduous canines, as well as between the canines and lower deciduous first molars;

- **Absence of spacing**: the teeth in the anterior segment had interproximal contacts. In these arches, there was an absence of interincisor and primate spaces, bilaterally;

- **Crowding**: in addition to the absence of interdental spaces, one or more deciduous teeth were deviated buccally and/or lingually in relation to their respective alveolar processes.

Considering the opinion of some authors (BAUME, 1950; EL-NOFELY; SADEK; SOLIMAN, 1989), who recognize interdental spaces in the deciduous dentition as characteristics related to congenital traits, as well as the observation by Zadik, Stern and Litner (1977) regarding the association between anterior spacing and non-nutritive sucking habits, it is suggested that these deleterious habits are probably associated with the widening of spaces. It would therefore be important to evaluate another occlusal characteristic that is related to non-nutritive sucking habits and widens the available space in the anterior segment of the dental arch. The most frequent occlusal alteration that is possibly associated with anterior spacing in the upper arch is increased overjet. Various researchers have pointed to the high prevalence of this occlusal alteration in children with non-nutritive sucking habits (ADAIR *et al.*, 1995; BISHARA *et al.*; 2006; ITO, 2006; SERRA-NEGRA; PORDEUS; ROCHA JR., 1997; WARREN *et al.*, 2001).

The overjet, also known as the horizontal interincisor gap, corresponded to the distance in millimeters between the buccal surface of the lower central incisors and the incisal edges of the upper central incisors, with the teeth in the MIH position. The measurement was quantified using a millimeter ruler (Morelli® , Sorocaba, SP) parallel to the occlusal plane.

Based on these measurements, the overshoot was classified as follows (FIGURE 4.1):

■ *Negative* (anterior crossbite): the lower deciduous central incisors are located in a buccal position to the upper deciduous central incisors, characterizing a negative horizontal crossbite;

■ *Null*: the horizontal distance between the upper and lower incisal edges is zero;

■ *Normal*: the horizontal distance between the upper and lower incisal edges does not exceed 2 mm;

■ *Increased*: horizontal distance between upper and lower incisal edges greater than 2 mm.

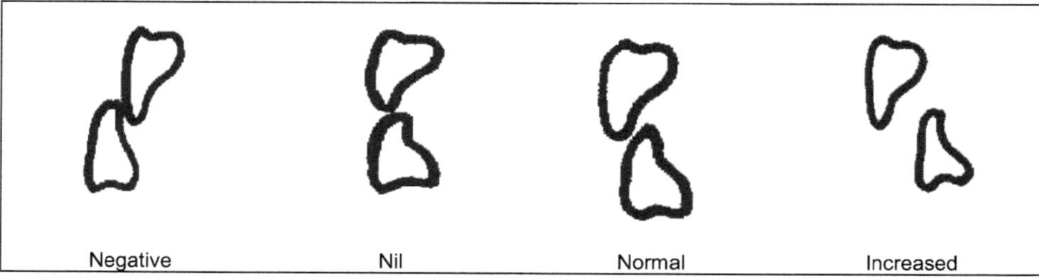

Figure 4.1 - Types of spares

4.4 Inclusion criteria

The children included in the samples met the criteria:

- Questionnaires answered properly;

- Complete deciduous dentition, with no erupted or erupting permanent teeth;

- Absence of extensive caries lesions, coronal destruction or proximal restorations that caused changes in the mesio-distal width of the teeth;

- No early loss of deciduous teeth;

- Absence of dental anomalies in terms of shape, number, structure and eruption;

- No cleft lip or palate syndromes;

- Never undergone orthodontic and/or speech therapy treatment.

4.5 Study groups

In the comparative evaluations of anterior interdental spacing characteristics in the upper and lower arches, the samples of Japanese-Brazilians and leucoderms were analyzed by age group and sex. However, in order to analyze the possible effects of non-nutritive sucking habits and increased overjet on the characteristics of *generalized anterior spacing* or *only the presence of primate spaces in* the upper arch, Japanese-Brazilians and Caucasians were separated into two groups according to the history of these deleterious habits (ITO, 2006):

- Control: children with no history of non-nutritive sucking habits;

- Suckers: children who exhibited non-nutritive sucking habits (finger sucking and/or pacifier sucking) at the time of the clinical assessment or had stopped doing so in the last twelve months.

The subdivision into age groups, as well as by gender, was not maintained in the analysis of the possible effects of non-nutritive sucking habits on occlusion, due to the relatively low frequency of sucking children.

4.6 Statistical treatment

4.6.1 Descriptive statistical analysis

The data collected was subjected to descriptive statistical analysis, with frequency distributions relating to the history of non-nutritive sucking habits and the occlusal characteristics under study according to age group and gender for each ethnic group.

4.6.2 Inferential statistical analysis

Next, the data on anterior interdental spacing characteristics were compared according to age group and gender for each ethnic group using Pearson's chi-square test. Multiple logistic regression models were used to analyze the effects of age group (2-4 years and 5-6 years), sex (male and female) and ethnic group (Caucasian and Japanese-Brazilian) on the prevalence of each of the characteristics related to anterior interdental spacing in the upper and lower arches. To assess the association between the occlusal characteristics *generalized anterior spacing* or *just the presence of primate spaces* in the upper arch and non-nutritive sucking habits, a multiple logistic regression model was also fitted, because another factor included in this analysis was increased overjet. For this last analysis, the characteristics *generalized anterior spacing* or *only* the *presence of primate spaces* were selected because they implied an increase in the space available in the anterior segment of the dental arches. The pre-established significance level was 5%.

Multiple logistic regression models allow the effects of more than one co-variable to be investigated simultaneously and provide *odds ratios* (OR). The OR value expresses the association between the characteristic in question and the co-variables studied.

5 RESULTS

5.1 Distribution of anterior interdental spacing characteristics in

Japanese-Brazilians

Graph 5.1 shows the distribution of children according to sex in these age groups. Boys predominated in the 2-4 age group (54.1%). Girls represented a much higher percentage than boys in the 5-6 age group (57.4%).

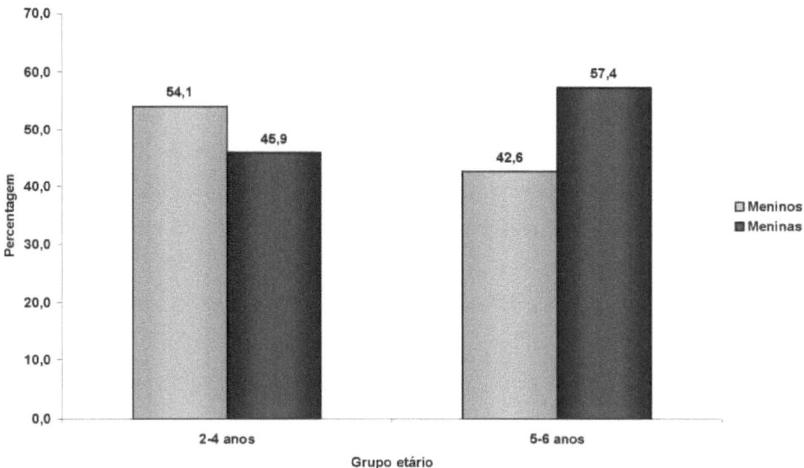

Graph 5.1 - Distribution of the Japanese-Brazilian sample by sex in the age groups.

Table 5.1 shows the absolute and percentage distribution of the characteristics surveyed in the upper and lower arches. The most prevalent feature was generalized spacing in the upper (46.2%) and lower (53.3%) arches. It should be noted that primate spaces were more frequent in the upper arch than in the lower arch (28.2% *versus* 15.3%). The values for the prevalence of crowding were very close in both arches, ranging from 4.0% to 4.9%.

Table 5.1 - Prevalence of anterior interdental spacing characteristics by arch in the Japanese-Brazilian sample.

Features	Upper arch		Lower arch	
	n	%	n	%
absent	88	21,7	107	26,4
primate spaces	114	28,2	62	15,3
generalized	187	46,2	216	53,3

33

| crowding | 16 | 4,0 | 20 | 4,9 |
| Total | 405 | 100,0 | 405 | 100,0 |

5.1.1 Evaluation of anterior interdental spacing characteristics according to age group and gender in a sample of Japanese-Brazilians

It was hypothesized that studying more diverse age groups (2-3 years, 4 years and 5-6 years) could provide detailed information on changes in the prevalence of the characteristics studied. However, despite the percentage differences, these were not statistically significant (APPENDIX C). Thus, the statistical analyses were carried out considering the two age groups proposed in the study design.

Graphs 5.2 and 5.3 show the prevalence of anterior spacing characteristics by age group in the upper and lower arches, respectively. In the upper arch, it can be seen that the frequency of the *absent* characteristic was lower in the 5 to 6 age group (18.9%) than in the 2 to 4 age group (23.4%). On the other hand, generalized spaces were more prevalent in the 5 to 6 age group (49.3%) compared to the 2 to 4 age group (44.4%). In the lower arch, the frequency values were slightly different in the age groups studied and, in general, were not very different from those observed for the total sample (Table 5.1).

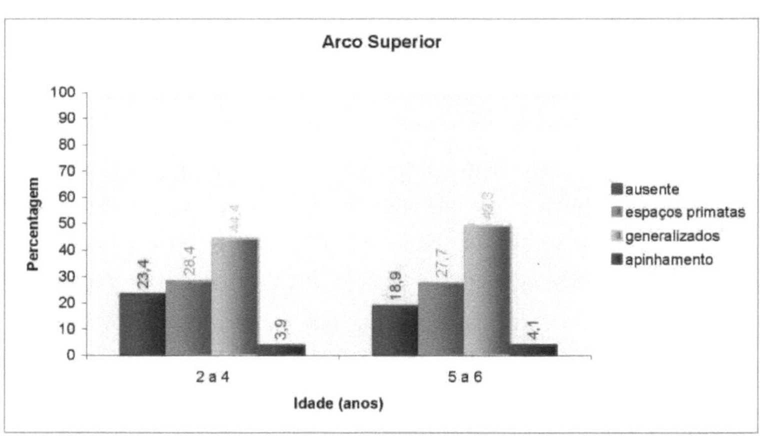

Graph 5.2 - Distribution of anterior spacing characteristics according to age group for the upper arch in Japanese-Brazilians.

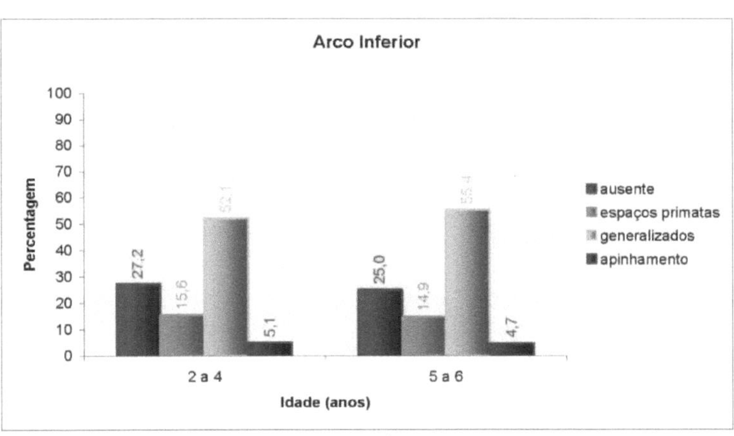

Graph 5.3 - Distribution of anterior spacing characteristics according to age group for the lower arch in Japanese-Brazilians.

Graphs 5.4 and 5.5 show the distribution of prevalence rates for anterior spacing characteristics in the upper arch for males and females, respectively. Considering the total sample as a parameter (Table 5.1), the percentage values obtained for both sexes were close. However, there were differences between the age groups for females and males. In the group of girls, the frequency of the *absent* characteristic was lower in the 5 to 6 age group (16.5%) than in the 2 to 4 age group (24.6%). However, generalized spaces were more prevalent in the 5 to 6 age group (51.8% *versus* 43.2%). Crowding was more frequent in the 2 to 4 age group (5.1%) compared to the 5 to 6 age group (2.4%). For the group of boys, the inverse behavior regarding the prevalence of crowding is interesting, with this characteristic being more prevalent in the 5 to 6 age group (6.4% *versus* 2.9%).

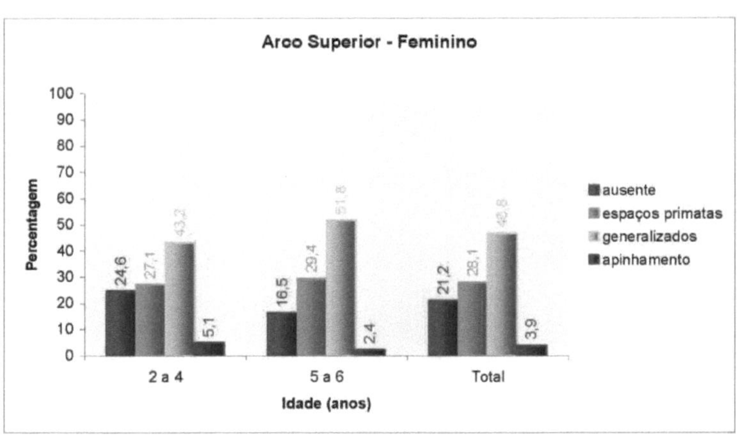

Graph 5.4 - Prevalence of anterior spacing characteristics in the upper arch, for females, in Japanese-Brazilians.

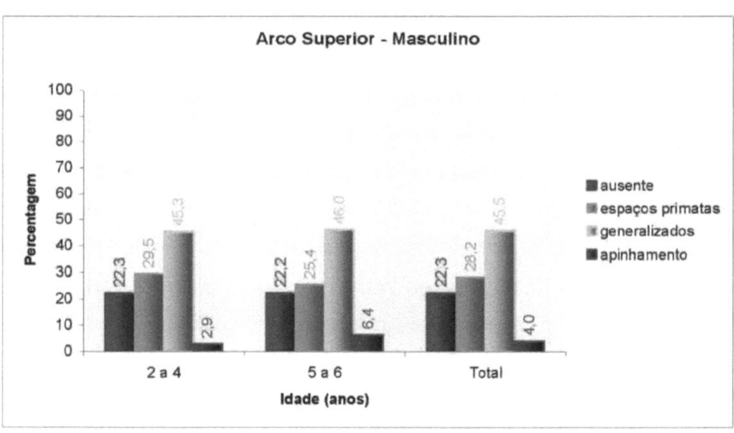

Graph 5.5 - Prevalence of anterior spacing characteristics in the upper arch, for males, in Japanese-Brazilians.

Graphs 5.6 and 5.7 show the frequencies of the anterior spacing characteristics in the lower arch for males and females, respectively. Taking into account the data from the total sample (Table 5.1), with the exception of the *crowding* characteristic, the percentage values obtained for the other variables in both sexes were different, but not excessively discrepant. In the group of girls, the frequency of generalized spaces was higher in the 5 to 6 age group (54.1%) than in the 2 to 4 age group (48.3%). Crowding was also more frequent in the 2 to 4 age group (6.8%) compared to the 5 to 6 age group (2.4%). For boys, the characteristics *absent* and *primate spaces were* less frequent in the older age

36

group. On the other hand, generalized spaces were more prevalent in the 5 to 6 age group (57.1% *versus* 55.4%). The opposite behavior remains with regard to the prevalence of crowding, which was more prevalent in the 5 to 6 age group (7.9% *versus* 3.6%).

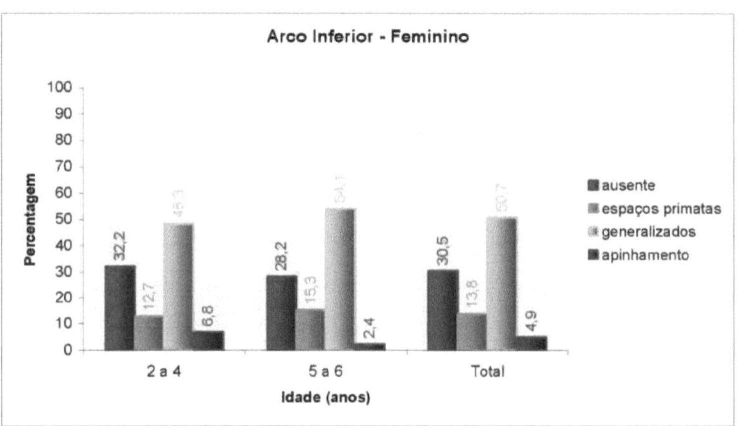

Graph 5.6 - Prevalence of anterior spacing characteristics in the lower arch, for females, in Japanese-Brazilians.

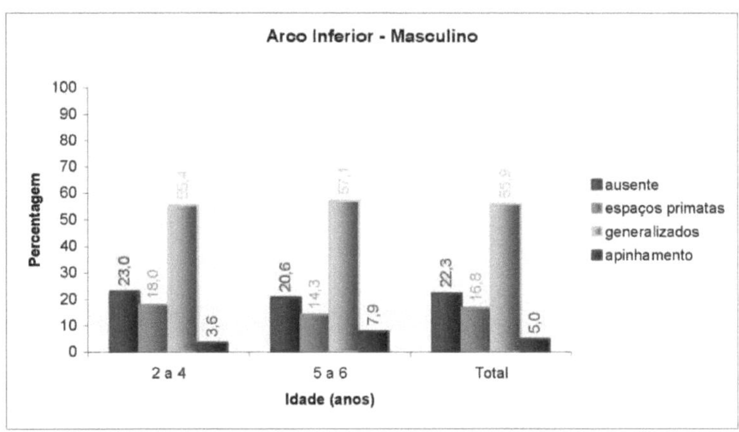

Graph 5.7 - Prevalence of anterior spacing characteristics in the lower arch, for males, in Japanese-Brazilians.

Pearson's chi-squared test ($a = 0.05$) was used to identify differences between the age groups and the sexes with regard to the prevalence of the characteristics studied in the upper and lower arches. Table 5.2 shows that there were no significant differences between the groups.

37

Table 5.2 - Frequency comparisons of anterior spacing characteristics between age groups and sexes, by dental arch, in Japanese-Brazilians.

Comparisons	Upper arch		Lower arch	
	λ^2	p-value	λ^2	p-value
age group	1,3717	0,712	0,4162	0,937
sex	0,0911	0,993	3,7421	0,291

5.2 Distribution of anterior interdental spacing characteristics in leucoderms

Graph 4.2 shows the distribution of children according to sex in these age groups. The presence of girls is predominant in both groups: 24 years (51.7%) and 5-6 years (52.2%). However, the disparities are not as striking as in the Japanese-Brazilian sample.

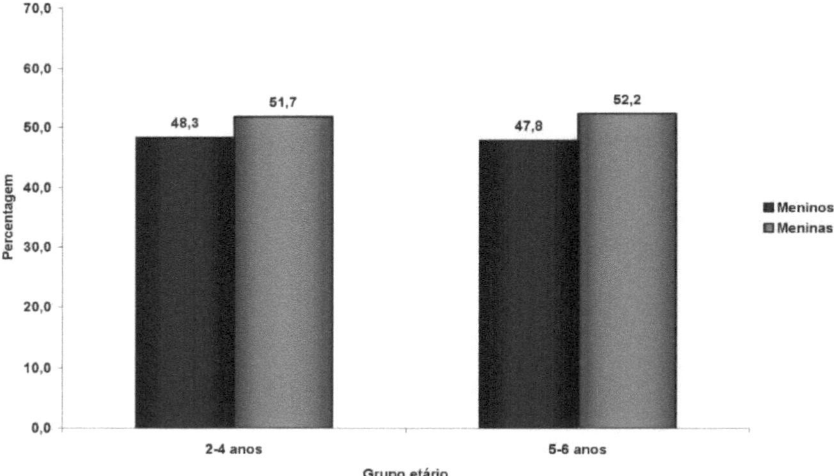

Graph 5.8 - Distribution of the leucoderm sample by sex in the age groups.

Table 5.3 shows the absolute and percentage distribution of the characteristics surveyed in the upper and lower arches. The most prevalent feature was generalized spacing in the upper (50.2%) and lower (51.4%) arches. Again, primate spaces were more frequent in the upper arch than in the lower arch (22.9% *versus* 12.6%). On the other hand, the prevalence of crowding was higher in the lower arch (12.8% *versus* 3.9%).

Table 5.3 - Prevalence of anterior interdental spacing characteristics by arch in the leucoderm sample.

Characteristic ■	Upper arch		Lower arch	
	n	%	n	%

absent	117	22,9	119	23,3
primate spaces	117	22,9	64	12,6
generalized	256	50,2	262	51,4
crowding	20	3,9	65	12,8
Total	510	100,0	510	100,0

5.2.1 Evaluation of anterior interdental spacing characteristics according to age group and sex, in a sample of Yucoderms

Graphs 5.9 and 5.10 show the prevalence of anterior spacing characteristics by age group in the upper and lower arches, respectively. In the upper arch, the frequencies obtained were similar to those observed for the total sample (Table 5.3). On the other hand, in the lower arch, generalized spaces were more prevalent in the 2 to 4 age group (55.8%) compared to the 5 to 6 age group (47.4%). Crowding was more frequent in children aged 5 to 6 (14.8% *versus* 10.4%).

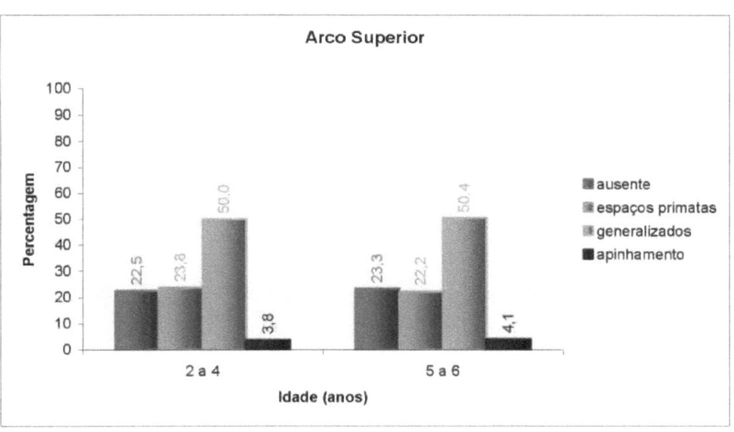

Graph 5.9 - Distribution of anterior spacing characteristics according to age group for the maxillary arch in leucoderms.

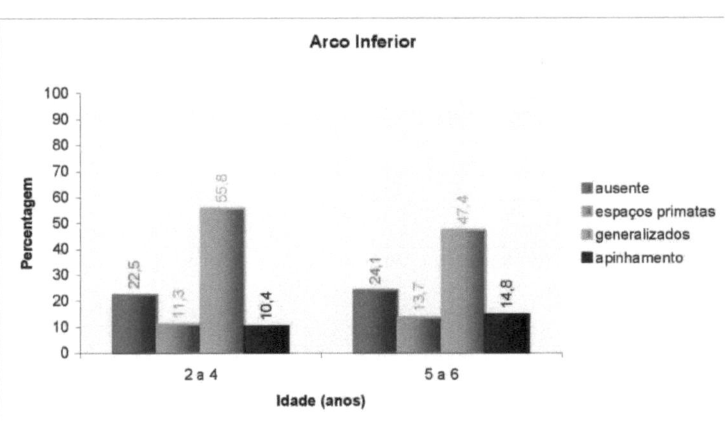

Graph 5.10 - Distribution of anterior spacing characteristics according to age group for the lower arch in leucoderms.

Graphs 5.11 and 5.12 show the distribution of prevalence rates for anterior spacing characteristics in the upper arch for males and females, respectively. Considering the total sample as a parameter (Table 5.3), the percentage values obtained for both sexes were slightly different. There were also differences between the age groups for females and males. In the group of girls, the frequency of the characteristic corresponding to generalized spaces was lower in the 5 to 6 age group (47.5%) than in the 2 to 4 age group (51.6%). Crowding was more frequent in the 5 to 6 age group (5.7%) compared to the 2 to 4 age group (3.2%). For the group of boys, the opposite was true with regard to the prevalence of crowding, which was more prevalent in the 2 to 4 age group (4.3% *versus* 2.3%), as well as generalized spaces, which were diagnosed more frequently in the 5 to 6 age group (53.5% *versus* 48.3%).

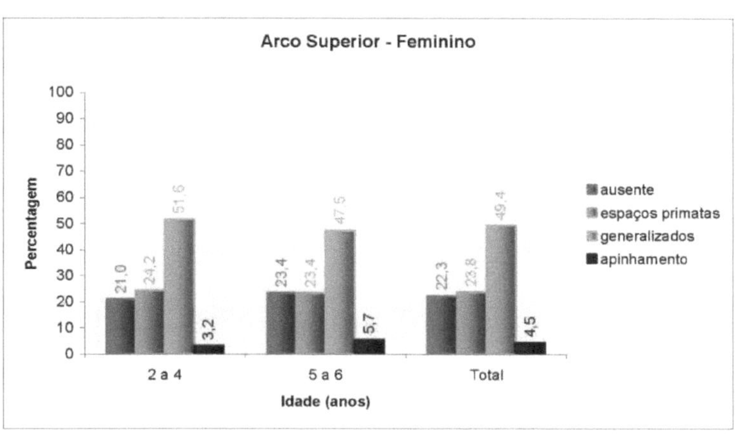

Graph 5.11 - Prevalence of anterior spacing characteristics in the upper arch for females in leucoderma.

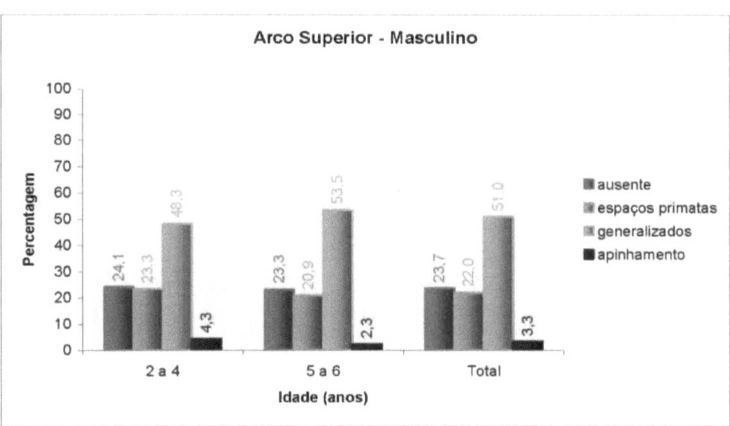

Graph 5.12 - Prevalence of anterior spacing characteristics in the upper arch, for males, in leucoderms.

Graphs 5.13 and 5.14 show the frequencies of anterior spacing characteristics in the lower arch for males and females, respectively. Taking into account the data from the total sample (Table 5.3), the percentage values obtained for both sexes were also generally different, but not excessively so. It is noteworthy that, in the group of girls, the frequency of generalized spaces was higher in the 2 to 4 age group (57.3%) than in the 5 to 6 age group (43.3%). Crowding, on the other hand, was more frequent in the 5 to 6 age group (18.4%) compared to the 2 to 4 age group (8.1%). Similarly, the prevalence of the *absent characteristic* was higher in the 5 to 6 age group (26.2% *versus* 22.6%). For boys, the

41

characteristics corresponding to generalized spaces and crowding showed lower frequencies in the more advanced age group. On the other hand, primate spaces were more prevalent in this group (15.5% *versus* 10.3%).

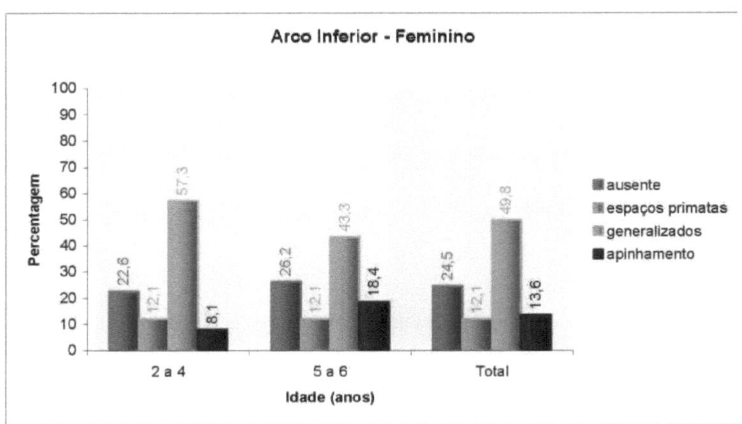

Graph 5.13 - Prevalence of anterior spacing characteristics in the lower arch for females in leucoderma.

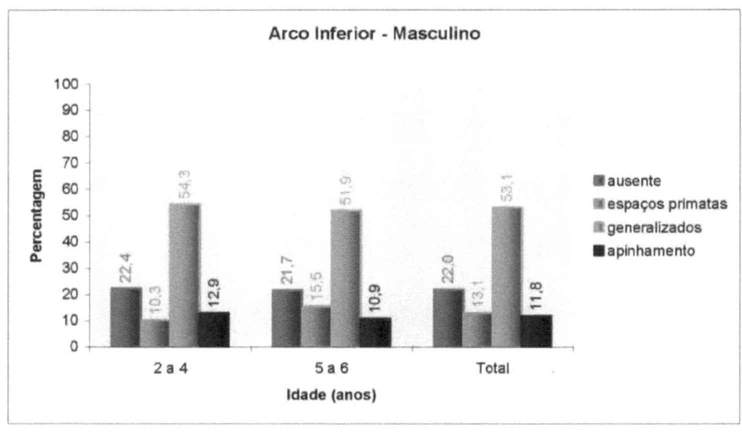

Graph 5.14 - Prevalence of anterior spacing characteristics in the lower arch for males in leucoderma.

Pearson's chi-squared test (a = 0.05) was used to identify differences between the age groups and the sexes with regard to the prevalence of the characteristics studied in the upper and lower arches. Table 5.4 shows that there were no significant differences between the groups.

Table 5.4 - Frequency comparisons of anterior spacing characteristics between age groups and sexes, by

42

dental arch, in leucoderms.

Comparisons	Upper arch		Lower arch	
	λ^2	p-value	λ^2	p-value
age group	0,2052	0,977	4,4289	0,219
sex	0,8585	0,835	1,0031	0,800

5.3 Multiple logistic regression models for the upper arch

Tables 5.5, 5.6, 5.7 and 5.8 show the logistic regression models for each of the anterior interdental spacing characteristics evaluated in the upper arch. The factors analyzed were: age group, gender and ethnic group. None of the models showed any significant factors. Therefore, there is no statistical evidence to indicate the effects of age, gender and race on the occlusal characteristics studied.

Table 5.5 - Multiple logistic regression model for the prevalence of the characteristic corresponding to the absence of interdental spaces in the upper arch.

	Upper Arc - No spaces						
Factors	no		yes		Logistic regression		
	n	%	n	%	OR	(I.C. 95%)	p-value
2-4 years	383	77,1	114	22,9			
5-6 years	327	78,2	91	21,8	0,93	(0,67 ; 1,27)	0,633
male	344	77,0	103	23,0			
female	366	78,2	102	21,8	0,93	(0,68 ; 1,27)	0,663
leucoderms	393	77,1	117	22,9			
Japanese-Brazilians	317	78,3	88	21,7	0,92	(0,67 ; 1,26)	0,605

Table 5.6 - Multiple logistic regression model for the prevalence of the characteristic *primate spaces* in the upper arch.

	Upper Arc - Primate spaces						
Factors	no		yes		Logistic regression		
	n	%	n	%	OR	(I.C. 95%)	p-value
2-4 years	367	73,8	130	26,2			
5-6 years	317	75,8	101	24,2	0,94	(0,67 ; 1,27)	0,673
male	336	75,2	111	24,8			

	348	74,4	120	25,6	1,05	(0,78 ; 1,42)	0,736
female	348	74,4	120	25,6	1,05	(0,78 ; 1,42)	0,736
leucoderms	393	77,1	117	22,9			
Japanese-Brazilians	291	71,9	114	28,1	1,30	(0,96 ; 1,76)	0,087

Table 5.7 - Multiple logistic regression model for the prevalence of the characteristic corresponding to generalized spaces in the upper arch.

	Upper Arc - Generalized spaces						
	no		yes		Logistic regression		
Factors	n	%	n	%	OR	(I.C. 95%)	p-value
2-4 years	263	52,9	234	47,1			
5-6 years	209	50,0	209	50,0	1,10	(0,84 ; 1,43)	0,485
male	230	51,5	217	48,5			
female	242	51,7	226	48,3	0,98	(0,76 ; 1,27)	0,893
leucoderms	254	49,8	256	50,2			
Japanese-Brazilians	218	53,8	187	46,2	0,86	(0,66 ; 1,13)	0,279

Table 5.8 - Multiple logistic regression model for the prevalence of the upper arch *crowding* characteristic.

Upper Arch - Crowding

	no		yes		Logistic regression		
Factors	n	%	n	%	OR	(I.C. 95%)	p-value
2-4 years	478	96,2	19	3,8			
5-6 years	401	95,9	17	4,1	1,06	(0,54 ; 2,09)	0,867
male	431	96,4	16	3,6			
female	448	95,7	20	4,3	1,20	(0,61 ; 2,35)	0,596
leucoderms	490	96,1	20	3,9			
Japanese-Brazilians	389	96,0	16	4,0	1,02	(0,52 ; 2,01)	0,953

5.4 Multiple logistic regression models for the lower arch

Tables 5.9, 5.10, 5.11 and 5.12 show the logistic regression analyses for each of the anterior interdental spacing characteristics evaluated in the lower arch. The factors analyzed were: age group, gender and ethnic group. The only model that showed any significant factor was the one adjusted for the prevalence of crowding. Only the race factor was significant (p = 0.000). According to Table 5.13, Caucasians were 2.81 times more likely to develop lower arch crowding than Japanese-Brazilians.

Table 5.9 - Multiple logistic regression model for the prevalence of the characteristic corresponding to the absence of interdental spaces in the lower arch.

| Lower Arch - No spaces | | | | | | | |
| Factors | no | | yes | | Logistic regression | | |
	n	%	n	%	OR	(I.C. 95%)	p-value
2-4 years	373	75,1	124	24,9			
5-6 years	316	75,6	102	24,4	0,98	(0,72 ; 1,34)	0,912
male	348	77,9	99	22,1			
female	341	72,9	127	27,1	1,31	(0,97 ; 1,78)	0,077
leucoderms	391	76,7	119	23,3			
Japanese-Brazilians	298	73,6	107	26,4	1,18	(0,87 ; 1,61)	0,282

Table 5.10 - Multiple logistic regression model for the prevalence of the characteristic *primate spaces* in the lower arch.

| Lower arch - Primate spaces | | | | | | | |
| Factors | no | | yes | | Logistic regression | | |
	n	%	n	%	OR	(I.C. 95%)	p-value
2-4 years	430	86,5	67	13,5			
5-6 years	359	85,9	59	14,1	1,11	(0,76 ; 1,63)	0,597
male	381	85,2	66	14,8			
female	408	87,2	60	12,8	0,85	(0,58 ; 1,24)	0,390
leucoderms	446	87,5	64	12,5			
Japanese-Brazilians	343	84,7	62	15,3	1,28	(0,87 ; 1,87)	0,208

Table 5.11 - Multiple logistic regression model for the prevalence of the characteristic corresponding to generalized spaces in the lower arch.

| Lower Arc - Generalized spaces | | | | | | | |
| Factors | no | | yes | | Logistic regression | | |
	n	%	n	%	OR	(I.C. 95%)	p-value
2-4 years	229	46,1	268	53,9			

Factor	n	%	n	%	OR	(I.C. 95%)	p-value
5-6 years	208	49,8	210	50,2	0,88	(0,67 ; 1,14)	0,334
male	204	45,6	243	54,4			
female	233	49,8	235	50,2	0,85	(0,66 ; 1,11)	0,232
leucoderms	248	48,6	262	51,4			
Japanese-Brazilians	189	46,7	216	53,3	1,06	(0,81 ; 1,38)	0,687

Table 5.12 - Multiple logistic regression model for the prevalence of the characteristic lower arch *crowding*.

	Lower Arch - Crowding						
	no		yes		Logistic regression		
Factors	n	%	n	%	OR	(I.C. 95%)	p-value
2-4 years	459	92,4	38	7,6			
5-6 years	371	88,8	47	11,2	1,33	(0,84 ; 2,09)	0,227
male	408	91,3	39	8,7			
female	422	90,2	46	9,8	1,11	(0,71 ; 1,75)	0,640
leucoderms	445	87,3	65	12,7			
Japanese-Brazilians	385	95,1	20	4,9	0,37	(0,22 : ; 0,63)	0,000

Table 5.13 - Logistic regression model for the prevalence of the characteristic lower arch *crowding*, considering only ethnic group.

	Lower Arch - Crowding					
	no		yes		Logistic regression	
Ethnic group	n	%	n	%	OR (I.C. 95%)	p-value
Japanese-Brazilians	385	95,	120	4,9		
leucoderms	445	87,	365	12,7	2,81 (1,67 ; 4,72)	0,000

To confirm the results of the logistic regression models and check for differences in the prevalence of spacing characteristics between the sexes and age groups, Pearson's chi-squared test with Bonferroni correction for multiple comparisons was applied (APPENDIX D). Assuming a significance level of 5% for the total set of comparisons, each individual test was evaluated at a significance level of 0.625% (5%/8 - where 8 is the total number of tests).

5.5 Analysis of non-nutritive sucking habits and increased overjet as factors affecting the prevalence of anterior interdental spaces in the upper arch

In this part of the analysis, only children who had never shown non-nutritive sucking habits (thumb sucking and/or pacifier sucking) and those who still showed habits or had discontinued them no more than 12 months before the date of the clinical examination were included. The sample was reduced to 469 children (without distinguishing between Japanese and Brazilian), 391 of whom belonged to the control group - without habits (83.3%) and 78 to the group of suckers (16.7%). Table 5.14 shows the distribution of this sub-sample according to the presence or absence of non-nutritive sucking habits (as described above), by ethnic group. It should be noted that in the leucoderm group, the percentage of suckers is twice as high compared to the Japanese-Brazilians.

Table 5.14 - Distribution of the sub-sample selected according to the history of non-nutritive sucking habits, by ethnic group.

| Ethnic group | Non-nutritive sucking habits | | | | Total | |
| | Control | | Suction units | | | |
	n	%	n	%	n	%
leucoderms	167	42,7	52	66,7	219	46,7
Japanese-Brazilians	224	57,3	26	33,3	250	53,3
Total	391	100,0	78	100,0	469	100,0

Controls: no history of non-nutritive sucking habits.

Suckers: had habits or discontinued them no more than 12 months ago.

Graphs 5.15 and 5.16 show the distribution of the sub-sample according to the presence or absence of increased overjet and the history of non-nutritive sucking habits, in leucoderms and Japanese-Brazilians, respectively. It was observed that among leucoderms, there was a higher frequency of children with increased overjet (31.1% *versus* 15.2%). Among the leucoderms with increased overjet, 27% were in the control group and 44.2% in the suction group, while among the Japanese-Brazilians, the respective percentages were 13.4% and 30.8%.

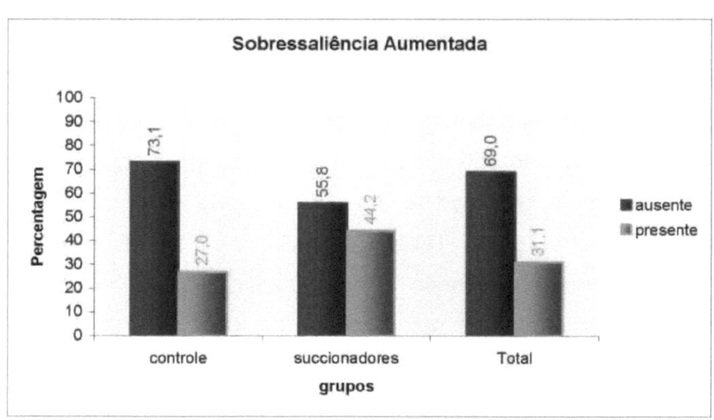

Graph 5.15 - Distribution of leucodermic children according to the presence of increased overjet and a history of pacifier and/or finger sucking habits (*Control: children with no history of non-nutritive sucking habits*)

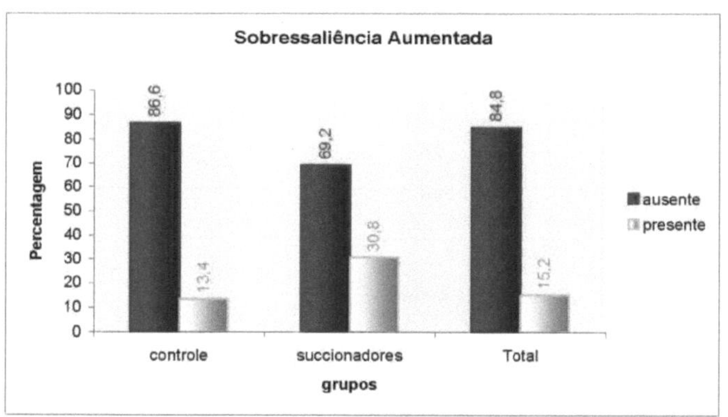

Graph 5.16 - Distribution of Japanese-Brazilian children according to the presence of increased overjet and a history of pacifier and/or finger sucking habits (*Control: children with no history of non-nutritive sucking habits*)

In order to evaluate the frequencies of generalized anterior spacing or primate spaces in the upper arch in relation to the presence of increased overjet, Graphs 5.17 and 5.18 were produced. The percentages of these two characteristics are high in leucoderms and Japanese-Brazilians (approximately 72%), which corroborates the relatively high frequency of anterior spaces in the deciduous dentition. In addition, it was found that in children with increased overjet, there is a higher prevalence of the aforementioned occlusal characteristics, both in leucoderms (77.9% *versus* 69.5%) and in Japanese-Brazilians (79% *versus* 71.7%). However, the logistic regression analysis showed no effect of increased overjet or non-nutritive sucking habits on the prevalence of generalized anterior spacing or primate spaces in the upper arch (Table 5.15).

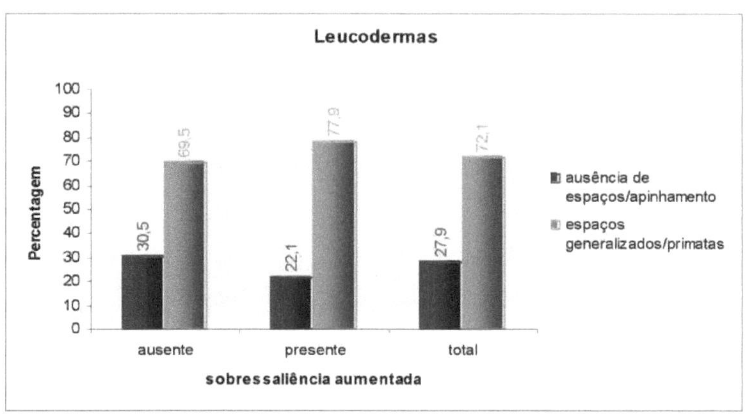

Graph 5.17 - Distribution of leucoderma children according to the presence of generalized anterior spaces or primate spaces in the upper arch and increased overjet.

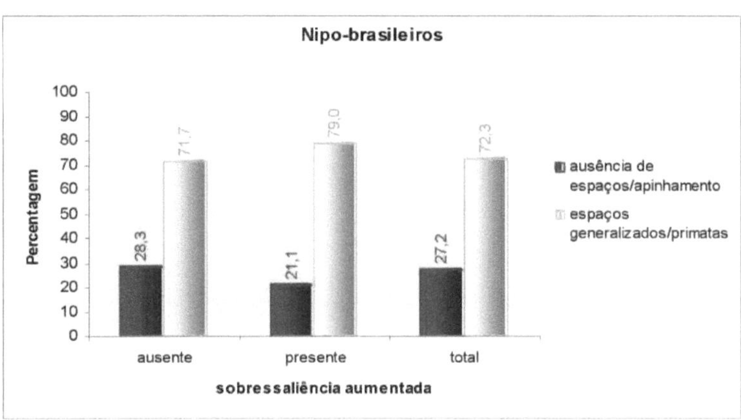

Graph 5.18 - Distribution of Japanese-Brazilian children according to the presence of generalized anterior spaces or primate spaces in the upper arch and increased overjet.

Table 5.15 - Logistic regression model for the frequency of generalized spacing or primate spaces in the upper arch as a function of increased overjet and history of non-nutritive sucking habits.

| Factors | Generalized anterior spacing / primate spaces | | | | | | |
| | no | | yes | | Logistic regression | | |
	n	%	n	%	OR	(I.C. 95%)	p-value

Over-emphasis increased	no	106	29,2	257	70,8			
	yes	23	21,7	83	78,3	1,42	(0,84; 2,39)	0,186
Non-nutritive sucking habits	control	112	28,6	279	71,4			
	suction units	17	21,8	61	78,2	1,35	(0,75; 2,43)	0,324

6 DISCUSSION

6.1 Considerations on the ethnic groups studied

Brazil's vast geography and, consequently, the diversity of ethnic, behavioral and sociocultural characteristics of its population groups, support and motivate the development of comparative studies on a series of epidemiological indicators. Considering oral health as an important axis of general health, assessing the occlusal patterns of different Brazilian ethnic groups is not only interesting, but also useful from a clinical point of view. Several national and foreign researchers have undertaken comparative investigations into occlusal characteristics in the deciduous dentition. Some of these studies are mentioned below.

Kerosuo (1990) observed that melanoderm children had a significantly lower rate of dental crowding compared to Finnish children of Caucasian origin. In Finnish children, pacifier sucking was quite common (77%). With regard to the lower frequency of crowding in melanoderms, this finding was later confirmed by Anderson (2007). In a comparative study involving measurements of the width, length and perimeter of the dental arch, as well as the quantification of interdental spaces, this researcher found that the dimensions analyzed were significantly greater in African-Americans than in American children of European descent.

After analyzing values for the mean-distal diameters of the crowns of deciduous teeth, Kuswandari and Nishino (2004) mentioned that Javanese Indonesian children were similar to Hong Kong Chinese and Australian Aborigines. Caglar *et al.* (2005), in their multicenter study, pointed out that there were big differences in the prevalence of various malocclusions in the countries studied.

To show data from the same foreign country with marked ethnic traits, we can present the work of Onyeaso (2006), who examined children from the three largest ethnic groups in Nigeria (Yoruba, Ibo and Hausa). Interincisor spacing was more frequent in Ibo children (48.4%) and less diagnosed in Hausa (19.8%), p < 0.001. The distribution of bilateral primate spaces also showed significant differences for the lower arch, being more prevalent in the Ibo (49.4%) than in the Hausa (21.3%) and Yoruba (29.3%), p < 0.001. Highly significant ethnic differences were revealed for spacing characteristics.

When it comes specifically to Brazilian children, two studies have presented information on dental crowding in the deciduous dentition. Thomaz *et al.* (2002), based on a study involving four cities in the northeast of Brazil, found significantly higher rates of crowding in

Recife - PE and Bayeux - PB compared to Joao Pessoa - PB and Aracaju - SE. In the city of Sao Luis - MA, also in the north-east of Brazil, Thomaz and Valença (2005) found that children from rural areas were less likely to be crowded than those from urban areas.

The origin of the Japanese people is uncertain, but it is believed that they are the result of the miscegenation of various races and that, over the millennia, they emerged as a homogeneous population - with a common language, culture and group consciousness (REISCHAUER, 1980). The Japanese have therefore become an ethnic group. The state of Sao Paulo is home to the vast majority of Japanese descendants, approximately 76% of all residents in Brazil (MENGUE *et al.*, 2004). This high indicator justifies the development of comparative epidemiological studies with members of this population who, because they were born in Brazil and have a strong Japanese genetic heritage (50% ancestry), are called Japanese-Brazilians. In fact, research has already been carried out on the occlusal characteristics of Japanese-Brazilians (ITO, 2006; MENGUE *et al.*, 2004; SATO, 2006). However, a detailed evaluation of anterior interdental spacing characteristics in the deciduous dentition has not yet been made public. Furthermore, if interdental spacing did not represent an important aspect of occlusion, there would be no classic early works (BAUME, 1950; FOSTER; HAMILTON, 1969; MOORREES; CHADHA, 1965) or more current ones (ANDERSON, 2007; ONYEASO, 2006, FERREIRA *et al.*, 2005).

In order to compare the results obtained with the evaluations of Japanese-Brazilians, a sample group of leukoderma children was selected from the epidemiological collection of the Universidade Cidade de Sao Paulo - UNICID. Although this sample is racially mixed and is influenced by the same socio-cultural factors as the rest of the children registered in the collection (black, brown and yellow), it was chosen because it is a group that contains a reasonable number of members and has one racial characteristic: white skin color. Authors such as Moorrees and Chadha (1965), Kerosuo (1990), Rossato and Martins (1993, 1994) and Anderson (2007) have also assessed leucoderma children.

6.2 Comparative study of anterior interdental spacing characteristics

In both the Japanese-Brazilian and Leucoderma samples, the presence of generalized spaces in the upper and lower arches was the most prevalent feature. In Japanese-Brazilians, the frequencies were 46.2% in the upper arch and 53.3% in the lower arch. For leucodermas, the respective percentages were 50.2% and 51.4%. This finding is in line with the results of other studies (ABU ALHAIJA; QUDEIMAT, 2003; BAUME, 1950; EL-NOFELY; SADEK; SOLIMAN, 1989; FERREIRA *et al.*, 2005; KABUE; MORACHA; NG'ANG'A; 1995; OTUYEMI *et al.*, 1997; SILVA-FILHO *et al.*, 2002). However, the prevalence rates show remarkable variability - for the upper arch, from 86.65% in the study by Silva-Filho *et al.* (2002) to 37.7% in the study by Otuyemi *et al.* (1997); and for the lower arch, from 79.96% to 44%, also in the aforementioned scientific investigations. The data that is closest to that obtained in the present study is that of El-Nofely, Sadek and Soliman (1989), with Egyptian children. Presumably, the difference in percentages is due to methodological differences, including the examination of anterior interdental spacing, and the characteristics of the sample groups studied.

The second most frequent characteristic in the ethnic groups in this study would be the presence of primate spaces, specifically in the upper arch compared to the lower arch, in the samples of Japanese-Brazilians (28.2% *versus* 15.3%) and leucoderms (22.9% *versus* 12.6%). If, in addition to these frequencies, we look at the data presented in the previous paragraph, we can admit that the results of this study agree with those of Moorrees and Chadha (1965), Kabue, Moracha and Ng'ang'a (1995), Otuyemi *et al.* (1997), Soviero, Bastos and Souza (1999), Abu Alhaija and Qudeimat (2003), Carvalho and Valença (2004) and Anderson (2007), who *showed prevalence rates for primate spaces in more than 60% of the* samples. The explanation lies in the aggregation of percentage values. Considering that, during the clinical examination, a dental arch could be diagnosed as having generalized spacing if only one of the interdental spaces evaluated was absent, the children with arches that showed generalized spacing had at least one of the primate spaces.

The results of this study are corroborated by those of El-Nofely, Sadek and Soliman (1989) and Ferreira *et al.* (2005), who used a similar classification during diagnosis, considering dental arches that exhibited only primate spaces, and observed much higher percentage values of this characteristic in the maxilla. The distribution and frequency of interdental spaces in the anterior segment is quite variable (JOSHI; MAKHIJA, 1984; OTUYEMI *et al.*, 1997; SOVIERO; BASTOS; SOUZA, 1999). However, due to their constancy, primate spaces have become a peculiar feature of the deciduous dentition. Primate spaces are described as a genetic trait that is expressed in the deciduous dentition (BAUME, 1950; EL-NOFELY; SADEK; SOLIMAN, 1989). The frequency and width of primate spaces are said to be greater than for other diastemas (JOSHI; MAKHIJA, 1984; OTUYEMI *et al.*, 1997; SOVIERO; BASTOS; SOUZA, 1999). Anterior spacing and, more specifically, primate spaces are independent characteristics and may be present or not, associated or isolated in the upper or lower dental arches (FERREIRA *et al.*, 2001; PACE; CHELLOTI, 1981). Foster and Hamilton (1969), Joshi and Makhija (1984) and Soviero, Bastos and

Souza (1999) pointed out that primate spaces were more frequent bilaterally.

The absence of interdental spaces, although less common, is not a finding that characterizes abnormality in the deciduous dentition. In this study, the frequency of arches with absent interdental spaces ranged from 21.7% to 26.4% in Japanese-Brazilians and 22.9% to 23.3% in Caucasians; the highest percentages were observed for the lower arches. Similarly, Foster and Hamilton (1969), El-Nofely, Sadek and Soliman (1989) and Otuyemi *et al.* (1997) found a higher prevalence of absent interdental spaces in the lower arch. With regard to this characteristic, the comparative assessment with other studies (ABU ALHAIJA; QUDEIMAT, 2003; ALEXANDER; PRABHU, 1998; BAUME, 1950; JOSHI; MAKHIJA, 1984; OTUYEMI *et al.*, 1997; RAVN, 1975) is made difficult by the grouping of two variables: absence of interdental spaces and crowding.

In the present study, it was decided to segregate the aforementioned variables because several authors have pointed to crowding in the deciduous dentition as a deviation from clinically satisfactory occlusion (OVSENIK, FARCNIK, VERDENIK, 2004; THILANDER *et al.* 2001; THOMAZ *et al.*, 2002; THOMAZ; VALENÇA, 2005). In addition, there is scientific evidence based on longitudinal studies to support the proservation of children with crowding in the deciduous dentition as a valid course of action, with the aim of detecting and intercepting the reflexes in the mixed and permanent dentitions at an early stage (BISHARA; JAKOBSEN, 2006; ROSSATO; MARTINS, 1993).

Dental crowding can be defined as a discrepancy in the proportion between the width of the teeth and the size of the bone bases, which results in overlapping and rotation of the teeth (TSAI, 2003). The etiology is multifactorial (ALEXANDER; PRABHU, 1998), with crowding being influenced by genetic and environmental factors (TSAI, 2003). According to Tsai (2003), three conditions may be related to crowding in the deciduous dentition: excessively wide teeth, very narrow bone bases or a combination of both. Some authors have suggested that the perimeter measurement is not the factor that differentiates dental arches with and without anterior spacing (DINELLI; MARTINS; PINTO, 2004; EL-NOFELY; SADEK; SOLIMAN, 1989; TSAI, 2003). van der Linden (1974) explained that, in the deciduous dentition, the growth of the apical bone bases is generally sufficient to allow the teeth to be aligned from the moment of eruption. In the permanent dentition, there is often a discrepancy between the perimeter available in the arch and the space required for proper alignment of the teeth.

The diameter of the dental arches (BAUME, 1950; DINELLI; MARTINS; PINTO, 2004; EL-NOFELY; SADEK; SOLIMAN, 1989; TSAI, 2003) and the mesio-distal width of the deciduous teeth (EL-NOFELY; SADEK; SOLIMAN, 1989; MELO; ONO; TAKAGI, 2001) have been identified as the measurements that would generate the significant differences. In a longitudinal study of Japanese subjects, Imai *et al.* (2006) observed that the mean mid-distal widths of the central and lateral incisors were significantly greater in the group with crowding ($p < 0.01$). However, the authors suggested that there is no clear relationship between the shape (based on mesio-distal and buccal-lingual measurements) and the arrangement of the lower incisors. It is interesting to note that the absence of interdental spaces and crowding in the deciduous dentition can be compensated for by dimensional and cephalometric changes in the permanent dentition (ROSSATO; MARTINS, 1994). Bishara, Khadivi and Jakobsen (1995) explained that changes in dentofacial structures are complex and the processes interact in such a way as to influence the relationship between teeth, dental arches and the face.

For leucoderms, as in the permanent dentition, the prevalence of crowding was found to be higher in the lower arch (12.8% versus 3.9%). This result is in line with that observed by Ferreira et al. (2005). Notably, in the Japanese-Brazilian sample, the values for the prevalence of dental crowding were very close, ranging from 4% in the upper arch to 4.9% in the lower arch. The difference between the two samples was confirmed by the logistic regression analysis (TABLES 5.12 and 5.13). Leucoderms were 2.8 times more likely to develop crowding in the lower arch compared to Japanese descendants.

There was no sexual dimorphism for anterior interdental spacing characteristics in Japanese-Brazilians and leucoderms (TABLES 5.2 and 5.4). When evaluating aspects related to anterior spacing, several authors also found no differences between boys and girls (ALEXANDER; PRABHU, 1998; CARVALHO; VALENÇA, 2004; DINELLI; MARTINS; PINTO, 2004; FERREIRA *et al.*, 2005; SILVA-FILHO *et al.*, 2002; THOMAZ *et al.*, 2002). However, other researchers have mentioned sexual dimorphism (ABU ALHAIJA; QUDEIMAT, 2003; ANDERSON, 2007; SOVIERO; BASTOS; SOUZA, 1999). Abu Alhaija and Qudeimat (2003) and Anderson (2007) found that primate spaces were significantly wider in boys than in girls. In addition, boys had a significantly higher frequency of primate spaces.

When it came to investigating possible changes in anterior spacing characteristics as age progressed, the statistical analyses showed no differences between the age groups (TABLES 5.2 and 5.4). Bearing in mind the proportions and based on the interpretation of Graphs 5.4 to 5.7, it can be seen that, in both males and females, the distribution of frequencies for the upper and lower arches in the age groups follows a trend in the

Japanese-Brazilian sample. In the leucoderma sample, this is only true for the upper arch (GRAPHS 5.11 to 5.14).

Soviero, Bastos and Souza (1999) observed that there was a significant decrease in the number of children presenting interdental spaces with advancing age, for both arches, suggesting a tendency for spaces to close. Carvalho and Valença (2004) found a significantly reduced frequency of primate spaces for the 4 to 6 age group (p < 0.05), compared to the group of children aged 2 to 4 years.

Kerosuo (1990) mentioned that the prevalence of crowding in the anterior region increased with age in leucodermic children (3-4 years - 5%; 5-6 years - 16%) and melanodermic children (3-4 years - 5%; 5-6 years - 9%). The results of the study carried out by Ferreira *et al.* (2005) indicated that the frequency of crowding in the lower arch was significantly higher in children aged 6. Based on the studies by Kerosuo (1990) and Ferreira *et al.* (2005), it was decided to divide the sample by age group, since in the second age group (5-6 years old) a possible influence of the initial eruption process of the first permanent molars on anterior spacing in the deciduous arches could be speculated. However, with regard to dental crowding, Thomaz *et al.* (2002) also showed no statistical difference between age groups.

Some of the results presented in this study should be interpreted with a degree of caution. To assess changes in anterior interdental spacing with age, longitudinal studies would be preferable.

Moorrees and Chadha (1965), Rossato and Martins (1993) and Imai et al. (2006). However, prospective longitudinal surveys require more time and are subject to the evasion of many of the sample members. In the case of the Japanese-Brazilian sample, the logistical demands are even more unfavorable, as children from 9 cities in the state of Sao Paulo were examined.

6.3 Association between the prevalence of anterior interdental spaces and non-nutritive sucking habits

In 1977, Zadik, Stern and Litner mentioned a possible association between the appearance of interdental spaces in the deciduous dentition and non-nutritive sucking habits. Considering that increased overjet is the most frequent occlusal alteration in children with non-nutritive sucking habits (ADAIR *et al.*, 1995; BISHARA *et al.;* 2006; ITO, 2006; SERRA-NEGRA; PORDEUS; ROCHA JR., 1997; WARREN *et al.*, 2001, SANTOS *et al..*, 2007) and which could be associated with anterior spacing, two factors were evaluated in relation to the prevalence of the two characteristics involving the presence of spaces, *generalized spacing* or *only primate spaces*: non-nutritive sucking habits and increased overjet.

In this evaluation, only children who had never had non-nutritive sucking habits (thumb sucking and/or pacifier sucking) and those who still had them or had discontinued them no more than 12 months before the date of the clinical examination were included. The maximum period of 12 months between the cessation of habits and the clinical examination would be critical, because beyond this interval, the probability of self-correction of the increased overjet would be very high. Another point to be clarified in this analysis would be the grouping of Japanese-Brazilians and leucodermans because, although non-nutritive sucking habits are frequently observed in the Brazilian population in general, they are not very prevalent in Japanese descendants (ITO, 2006; SATO, 2006). Furthermore, the two characteristics of anterior spacing mentioned above were not affected by the ethnic group factor.

After interpreting Graphs 5.17 and 5.18, it can be seen that children with increased overjet had a higher prevalence of *generalized spacing* or *primate spaces only*. However, neither a positive history of non-nutritive sucking habits nor increased overjet were statistically associated with a higher prevalence of these characteristics (TABLE 5.15). It appears that there is an association between a positive history of prolonged non-nutritive sucking habits and a higher frequency of increased overjet. However, sucking habits are not necessarily related to the appearance of anterior spaces in the deciduous arch. It is suggested, according to Baume (1950) and El-Nofely, Sadek and Soliman (1989), that this is actually a genetic trait.

When it comes to assessing interdental spaces, a weakness that could be pointed out in this investigation lies in visual inspection, rather than the application of a method that would allow quantitative recording of spacing, using measuring instruments directly in the mouth (AZNAR *et al.*, 2006; OVSENIK; FARCNIK; VERDENIK, 2004) or on plaster models (ABU ALHAIJA; QUDEIMAT, 2003; ANDERSON, 2007; BAUME, 1950; KUSWANDARI; NISHINO, 2004; MELO; ONO; TAKAGI, 2001; MOORREES; CHADHA, 1965; NYSTROM, 1981; ROSSATO; MARTINS, 1993). However, the rigor in assessing the ethicality of research projects has gradually increased, and some physical examination procedures and molding can be judged as invasive. Assuming the argument before the Ethics Committee and the approval of such methods, one must also consider the children's acceptance of being subjected to a physical examination with measuring instruments inserted in the mouth or molding, which cause discomfort. In addition, it is impractical to obtain plaster models of numerous sample groups, such as the one used by Romero (2007), of 1377 children, from which the leucoderms evaluated in this study were selected.

7   CONCLUSIONS

According to the results obtained, it can be concluded that:

☐ In the Japanese-Brazilian sample, generalized anterior interdental spacing was the most prevalent feature in the upper and lower arches. The frequency of primate spaces was higher in the upper arch. However, for the characteristics relating to the absence of interdental spaces and crowding, the variation between the percentages calculated for the upper and lower arches was relatively small;

☐ In the sample of Brazilian leucoderms, the frequencies of the characteristics relating to the absence of interdental spacing and the presence of primate spaces showed a distribution pattern similar to that observed in Japanese Brazilians. It should be noted that generalized anterior spacing was diagnosed in approximately 50% of the upper and lower dental arches. However, the prevalence of dental crowding was 3 times higher in the lower arch compared to the upper arch;

☐ In both samples under study, there were no significant differences between age groups (2-4 years and 5-6 years) or sexual dimorphism for anterior interdental spacing characteristics;

☐ Leucoderms were 2.8 times more likely to develop dental crowding in the lower arch compared to Japanese-Brazilians;

☐ There was no evidence of an association between the prevalence of generalized anterior spacing or just the presence of primate spaces in the upper arch and a positive history of non-nutritive sucking habits.

REFERENCES[1]

Abu Alhaija ESJ, Qudeimat MA. Occlusion and tooth/arch dimensions in the primary dentition of preschool Jordanian children. **Int J Paediatr Dent**. 2003 July; 13(4): 2309.

Adair SM, Milano M, Lorenzo I, Russel C. Effects of current and former pacifier use on the dentition of 24- to 59-month-old children. **Pediatr Dent**. 1995 Nov.-Dec.; 17(7): 437-44.

Alexander S, Prabhu NT. Profiles, occlusal plane relationships and spacing of teeth in the dentitions of 3 to 4 year old children. **J Clin Pediatr Dent**. 1998 Summer; 22(4): 329-34.

Anderson AA. The dentition and occlusal development in children of African American descent. **Angle Orthod**. 2007 May; 77(3): 421-9.

Aznar T, Galân AF, Marin I, Dominguez A. Dental arch diameters and relationships to oral habits. **Angle Orthod**. 2006 May; 76(3): 441-5.

Baume LJ. Physiological tooth migration and its significance for the development of occlusion: I. The biogenetic course of the deciduous dentition. **J Dent Res.** 1950 Apr.; 29(2): 123-32.

Bishara SE, Jakobsen JR. Individual variation in tooth-size/arch-length changes from the primary to permanent dentitions. **World J Orthod**. 2006 Summer; 7(2): 145-53.

Bishara SE, Khadivi P, Jakobsen JR. Changes in tooth size-arch length relationships from the deciduous to the permanent dentition: A longitudinal study. **Am J Orthod and Dentofacial Orthop**. 1995 Dec.; 108(6): 607-13.

Bishara SE, Warren JJ, Broffitt B, Levy SM. Changes in the prevalence of nonnutritive sucking patterns in the first 8 years of life. **Am J Orthod Dentofacial Orthop**. 2006 July; 130(1): 31-6.

Caglar E, Larsson E, Andersson EM, Hauge MS, Ogaard B, Bishara S *et al*. Feeding, artificial sucking habits, and malocclusions in 3-year-old girls in different regions of the world. **J Dent Child**. 2005 Jan.-Apr.; 72(1): 25-30.

Carvalho KL, Valença AMG. Prevalence of normal deciduous occlusion characteristics in children aged 2 to 6 years. **Pesq Bras Odontoped Clin Integr**. 2004 May-August; 4(2): 113-20.

Dinelli TCS, Martins LP, Pinto AS. Dimensional changes of dental arches in children between 3 and 6 years of age. **Rev Dent Press Ortodon Ortoped Facial**. 2004 Jul.-Aug.;

---

1 According to Vancouver style. Abbreviation for journals according to MEDLINE databases.

9(4): 60-7.

El-Nofely A, Sadek L, Soliman N. Spacing in the human deciduous dentition in relation to tooth size and dental arch size. **Arch Oral Biol**. 1989; 34(6): 437-41.

Ferreira RI, Barreira AK, Soares CD, Alves AC. Prevalence of normal occlusion characteristics in deciduous teeth. **Pesqui Odontol Bras**. 2001 jan.-mar.; 15(1): 23-8.

Ferreira RI, Scavone-Jr H, Castro RG, Nascimento MAS, Romero CC. Assessment of interdental spacing in the anterior segment of deciduous arches. **Rev Odontol Unicid**. 2005 May-Aug; 17(2): 101-10.

Foster TD, Hamilton MC. Occlusion in the primary dentition. Study of children at 2 1/2 to 3 years of age. **Br Dent J**. 1969 Jan.; 126(2): 76-9.

Guimaraes JR CH. **Analysis of the influence of natural breastfeeding time on the development of non-nutritive sucking habits in the deciduous dentition** [Dissertation]. Sao Paulo: Universidade Cidade de Sao Paulo; 2004.

Imai H, Kuwana R, Yonezu T, Yakushiji M. The relation between tooth shape ratio and incisor arrangement in Japanese children. **Bull Tokyo Dent Coll**. 2006 May; 47(2): 45-50.

Ito C. **Association between non-nutritive sucking habits and anteroposterior occlusal relationships in deciduous teeth in Japanese-Brazilians** [Dissertation]. Sao Paulo: Universidade Cidade de Sao Paulo; 2006.

Joshi MR, Makhija PG. Some observations on spacing in the normal deciduous dentition of 100 Indian children from Gujarat. **Br J Orthod**. 1984 Apr.; 11(2): 75-9.

Kabue MM, Moracha JK, Ng'ang'a PM. Malocclusion in children aged 3-6 years in Nairobi, Kenya. **East Afr Med J**. 1995 Apr.; 72(4): 210-2.

Kataoka DY, Scavone-Jr H, Vellini-Ferreira F, Cotrin-Ferreira FA, Sato VCB. Study of the anteroposterior relationship between the deciduous dental arches of Japanese-Brazilian children aged 2 to 6 years.**Rev Dent Press Ortodon Ortoped Facial**. 2006; 2(5): 83-92.

Kerosuo H. Occlusion in the primary and early mixed dentitions in a group of Tanzanian and Finnish children. **ASDC J Dent Child**. 1990 July-Aug.; 57(4): 293-98.

Kharbanda OP, Sidhu SS, Shukla DK, Sundaram KR. A study of the etiological factors associated with the development of malocclusion. **J Clin Pediatr Dent**. 1994 Winter; 18(2): 95-8.

Kuswandari S, Nishino M. The mesiodistal crown diameters of primary dentition in

Indonesian Javanese children. **Arch Oral Biol**. 2004 Mar.; 49(3): 217-22.

Leighton BC. The early signs of malocclusion. **Eur J Orthod**. 2007 Apr.; 29(Suppl. 1): i89-i95.

Melo L, Ono Y, Takagi Y. Indicators of mandibular dental crowding in the mixed dentition. **Pediatr Dent**. 2001 Mar.-Apr.; 23(2): 118-22.

Mengue OCC, Scavone-Jr. H, Ferreira RI, Cotrim-Ferreira FA, Carvalho PEG, Sesma N, *et al.* Prevalence of posterior crossbite in deciduous dentition in Japanese-Brazilian children. **Rev Odontol UNICID**. 2004 Sep.-Dec.; 16(3): 213-22.

Moorrees CFA, Chadha JM. Available space for the incisors during dental development: a growth study based on physiologic age. **Angle Orthod**. 1965 Jan.; 35(1): 12-22.

Nystrom M. Spacing during the complete deciduous dentition period in a series of Finnish children. **Proc Finn Dent Soc**. 1981; 77(4): 202-10.

Onyeaso CO. Occlusion in the primary dentition. Part 1: A preliminary report on comparison of antero-posterior relationships and spacing among children of the major Nigerian ethnic groups. **Odontostomatol Trop**. 2006 June; 29(114): 9-14.

Otuyemi OD, Sote EQ, Isiekwe MC, Jones SP. Occlusal relationships and spacing or crowding of teeth in the dentitions of 3-4-year-old Nigerian children. **Int J Paediatr Dent**. 1997 Sept.; 7(3): 155-60.

Ovsenik M, Farcnik FM, Verdenik I. Comparison of intra-oral and study cast measurements in the assessment of malocclusion. **Eur J Orthod**. 2004 June; 26(3): 273-7.

Pace RSG, Chelloti A. Frequency of distribution of primate spaces in children with type I and II arches. **Rev Fac Odontol Univ Sao Paulo**. 1981 Jan.-Jun.; 19(1): 53-62.

Ravn JJ. Occlusion in the primary dentition in 3-year-old children. **Scand J Dent Res**.1975 May; 83(3):123-30.

Reischauer EO. **Japan, the story of a nation**. 6th ed. Tokyo: Charles E. Tutle Co.; 1980.

Romero CC. **Association between breastfeeding and overbite changes in the deciduous dentition** [Dissertation]. Sao Paulo: Universidade Cidade de Sao Paulo; 2007.

Rossato C, Martins DR. Anterior spacing in the deciduous dentition and its relationship with crowding in the permanent dentition. A longitudinal study. **Ortodontia**. 1993 May-August; 26(2): 81-7.

Rossato C, Martins DR. Dimensional and cephalometric changes in young Brazilian leucoderms with and without anterior spacing in the deciduous dentition.

Longitudinal study from deciduous to permanent dentition. **Ortodontia**. 1994 May-August; 27(2): 19-30.

Santos DC, Scavone-Junior H, Ferreira RI, Garib DG, Vellini-Ferreira F. Association between pacifier sucking habit, terminal relationship of deciduous second molars and overjet. **Rev Odontol UNESP**. 2007; 36(2): 137-43.

Scavone-Junior H, Santos DC, Garib DG, Ferreira RI, Vellini-Ferreira F, Kobayashi HM. Association between non-nutritive sucking habits and the antero-posterior relationship between deciduous dental arches. *Rev Odontol UNICID*. 2005; 17(3): 221227.

Sato VCB. **Association between non-nutritive sucking habits, vertical clearance and the transverse relationship between deciduous dental arches in Japanese-Brazilians** [Dissertation]. Sâo Paulo: Universidade Cidade de Sâo Paulo; 2006.

Serra-Negra JMC, Pordeus IA, Rocha Jr. JF. Study of the association between breastfeeding, oral habits and malocclusions. **Rev Odontol Univ Sâo Paulo**. 1997; 11(2): 79-86.

Silva-Filho OG, Rego MVNN, Silva PRB, Silva FPL, Ozawa TO. Intra-arch relationship in the normal deciduous dentition: diastemas, absence of diastemas and crowding. **J Bras Ortodon Ortop Facial**. 2002 Nov.-Dec.; 7(42): 501-9.

Soviero VLM, Bastos EPS, Souza IPR. Deciduous dentition: study of the prevalence of interproximal spaces in Brazilian children. **Rev Odontol Univ Sâo Paulo**. 1999 Apr.-Jun.; 13(2): 159-65.

Thilander B, Pena L, Infante C, Parada SS, Mayorga C. Prevalence of malocclusion and orthodontic treatment need in children and adolescents in Bogotà, Colombia. An epidemiological study related to different stages of dental development. **Eur J Orthod**. 2001 Apr.; 23(2): 153-67.

Thomaz EBAF, Ely MR, Lira CC, Moraes ES, Valença AMG. Prevalence of upper incisor protrusion, deep overbite, premature tooth loss and crowding in deciduous teeth. **J Bras Odontopediatr Odontol Bebê**. 2002 Jul.-Aug.; 5(26): 276-82.

Thomaz EBAF, Valença AMG. Prevalence of malocclusion and factors related to its occurrence in preschool children in the city of Sâo Luis - MA - Brazil. **RPG Rev Pós-Grad**. 2005 Apr./Jun.; 12(2): 212-21.

Tsai HH. Dental crowding in primary dentition and its relationship to arch and crown dimensions. **J Dent Child**. 2003 May/Aug.; 70(2): 164-9.

van der Linden FPGM. Theoretical and practical aspects of crowding in the human dentition. **J Am Dent Assoc**. 1974 July; 89 (1): 139-53.

Vieira ACG, Scavone-Jr H, Nahas ACR, Vellini-Ferreira F, Cotrin-Ferreira FA, Valle Corotti KM, Quaglio CL. Study of the prevalence of interincisor vertical mismatch in the deciduous dentition in Japanese-Brazilian children. ***Rev Odontol UNICID***. 2004; 16(2): 149-158.

Warren JJ, Bishara SE, Steinbock KL, Yonezu T, Nowak AJ. Effects of oral habits' duration on dental characteristics in the primary dentition. **J Am Dent Assoc**. 2001 Dec.; 132(12): 1685-93.

Zadik D, Stern N, Litner M. Thumb- and pacifier-sucking habits. **Am J Orthod**. 1977 Feb.; 71(2): 197-201.

ANNEX

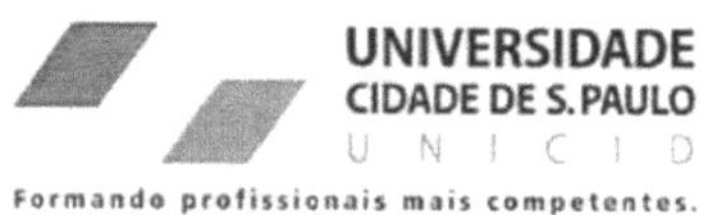

São Paulo, May 23, 2007.

I hereby declare for all intents and purposes that Research Protocol N^0 13259823 - **Association between Anterior Spacing and Pacifier Suction in Japanese-Brazilians and Leucoderms, in the Deciduous Dentition,** which has as researcher - Evandro Eloy Marcone Ferreira; was Submitted to the Research Ethics Committee of the Universidade Cidade de São Paulo and approved at a meeting on February 6, 2007.

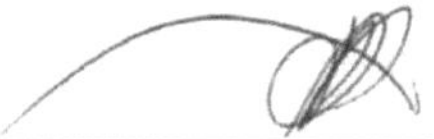

Prof. Dr. Clâudio Antonio Barbosa de Toledo President of CEP Universidade Cidade de São Paulo

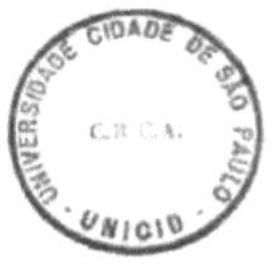

APPENDICES

APPENDIX A

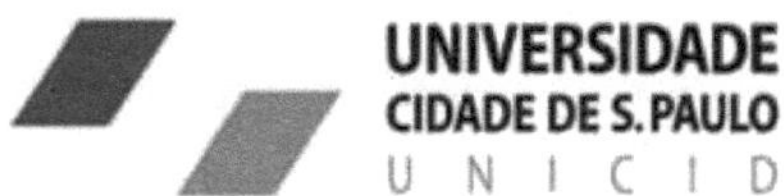

Dentistry course

Discipline of Orthodontics

Parents,

Inappropriate oral habits, such as prolonged use of pacifiers, bottles and thumb sucking, can cause changes in children's dental arches and speech. That's why we dentists would like to examine your child. Only after a clinical examination can we advise you on how to prevent and treat these changes at an early stage.

With the aim of making a diagnosis of the problems caused by inadequate oral habits, the Orthodontics Discipline team at the City University of Sao Paulo is working in municipal schools in the Tatuapé district. Our work involves 1. the authorization of parents for the dental evaluation of their children. Together with their consent, parents must answer a questionnaire about their children's oral habits;

2. The dental assessment of your children;

3. The response letter with the diagnosis of their children's oral health conditions;

4. Every Monday afternoon, from 2:30 to 4:00 p.m., a dentist specializing in orthodontics is available to answer questions at the City of Sao Paulo University Postgraduate Clinic.

Taking into account the importance of this work for children's oral health, we ask for your written authorization so that we can carry out the dental examination on your child during the school term and at the school itself.

I,   , R.G. _______________________________________ ,

I authorize the dental examination of my child by the Orthodontics Department of the City University of Sao Paulo.

Sao Paulo, _____ 2006 _____________ .

Signature: _______________________________

QUESTIONNAIRE FOR RESEARCHING INAPPROPRIATE HABITS

IDENTIFICATION AND GENERAL INFORMATION ABOUT THE FAMILY

1. Who is answering this questionnaire?

( ) The mother

( ) The father

( ) A relative

( ) Other responsible

2. Child's full name: _______________________________

3. Sex ( ) M ( ) F

4. Age: _______

5. Date of birth: ___/___/_________

6. School: EMEI _______________________________

7. Teacher: _______________________________

8. Living room: _______________________________

9. Period: ( ) Morning ( ) Intermediate ( ) Evening

10. Fill in the following information about the country, state and city where your child's family members were born:

Family	PAiS	STATE	CITY
Dad			
Mae			
Paternal grandfather			
Paternal grandmother			
Maternal grandfather			
Maternal grandmother			

11. Father's name: _______________________________

12. Level of education:

( ) First grade incomplete

( ) Completed primary school

( ) High school incomplete

( ) Completed high school

( ) Incomplete university degree

( ) Complete university degree

13. Mother's name: ____

14. Level of education:

( ) First grade incomplete

( ) Completed primary school

( ) High school incomplete

( ) Completed high school

( ) Incomplete university degree

( ) Complete university degree

15. Home address:

___Neighborhood: ________________ Zip code: __________

Phone: ____________________ Phone for messages: ________________

16. Number of children:

17. Adding up the salaries of all the people who work and help with household expenses, the total family income is:

( ) Less than R$ 300.00 per month

( ) From R$ 300.00 to R$ 600.00 per month

( ) From R$ 600.00 to R$ 1,200.00 per month

( ) From R$ 1,200.00 to R$ 1,800.00 per month

( ) From R$ 1,800.00 to R$ 2,400.00 per month

( ) More than R$ 2,400.00 per month

INFORMATION ABOUT THE CHILD'S HEALTH AND THE PRESENCE OF HABITS

18. Is your child currently undergoing medical treatment?

( ) Yes. Why? ____

( ) No

19. Has your child ever been examined by a dentist?

( ) Yes, when? _______________________________________

( ) No

20. Do you know what orthodontics is?

( ) Yes. What is it? _______________________________________

( ) No, but I'd like to know.

( ) No

21. Is your child undergoing speech therapy?

( ) Yes. Why? _______________________________________

( ) No, never.

( ) Not at the moment, but has been in treatment before.

22. Is your child undergoing orthodontic treatment?

( ) Yes. Why? _______________________________________

( ) No, never.

( ) Not at the moment, but has been in treatment before.

23. Mark the problem(s) your child has with an X:

( ) Visual impairment

( ) Hearing impairment

( ) Mental disability

( ) Cleft lip or lip-palate

( ) A syndrome. Which syndrome? _______________________________

( ) No such problems.

24. When drawing or writing, which hand does your child use more? ( ) right ( ) left ( ) can't answer

25. Has your child ever suffered an accident or trauma in the mouth? ( ) Yes. When?   . If any

consequence, please write.

____

( ) No

26.   Was your child breastfed?

( ) Yes ( ) No

27.   If your child was <u>breastfed,</u> how many months old was he or she weaned?

( ) Less than 3 months old

( ) He/she was between 3 and 6 months old

( ) He/she was between 6 and 9 months old

( ) He/she was between 9 and 12 months old (between 9 months and 1 year)

( ) More than 12 months old (more than 1 year old)

( ) I don't remember.

( ) He/she is still breastfeeding.

28.   If the child is still breastfeeding, the diet is supplemented with:

( ) Baby bottles

( ) Soups or homemade food. How many times a day?   _____________________

( ) Ready-made porridge. How many times a day? _______________

( ) Does not require complementary feeding.

29.   Has your child been or still is <u>only</u> bottle-fed?

( ) Yes

( ) No, never used a bottle.

30.   If the child uses or has used a bottle, please answer:

At what age did you <u>start</u> using? At what age did you <u>stop using</u>?

How many bottles a day until 1 year old? _______________

How many bottles a day until the age of 2?   _______________

How many bottles a day until the age of 3?   _______________

How many bottles a day until the age of 4?   _______________

How many bottles a day until the age of 5?   _______________

How many bottles a day until the age of 6? _________________

31. Does your child suck on a pacifier?

( ) Yes, he still sucks on a pacifier.

At what age did you start sucking on a pacifier?

( ) No, never sucked a pacifier.

( ) No. He used to suck a pacifier, but stopped.

At what age did he/she stop? How old was he/she when he/she started sucking on a pacifier?

32. When does or did your child suck on a pacifier?

( ) All day

( ) Sometimes. When? ____

( ) Just to sleep

Does he/she sleep or used to sleep through the night sucking on a pacifier? *( ) Yes ( ) No*

33. If your child sucks or has sucked on a pacifier, what kind?

( ) Ordinary pacifier

( ) Orthodontic pacifier

( ) Ordinary and orthodontic pacifiers

34. Does your child suck their thumb?

( ) Yes, he still sucks his thumb.

At what age did you start sucking your thumb?

( ) No, he's never sucked his thumb.

( ) No. He used to suck his thumb, but he stopped.

At what age did he/she stop? How old was he/she when he/she started sucking fingers?

35. When does or did your child suck their thumb(s)?

( ) All day

( ) Sometimes. When? ____

( ) Just to sleep

Does he/she sleep or used to sleep all night sucking his/her thumb(s)? *( ) Yes ( ) No*

36. Does your child have the habit of resting one hand on their face when watching TV or reading or studying?

( ) No, never had.

( ) He doesn't now, but he used to.

In this case, the habit started at what age?

And at what age was it stopped? ___________________

Which hand was used for support? ( ) right ( ) left

( ) Yes, currently has the habit.

In this case, at what age did the habit start?

Which hand is used for support? ( ) right ( ) left

37. Does your child sleep with one hand under their face?

( ) No

( ) No, but I used to sleep like this.

In this case, the habit started at what age?

And at what age was it stopped? ___________________

Which hand was used for support? ( ) right ( ) left

( ) Yes

In this case, at what age did the habit start?

Which hand is used for support? ( ) right ( ) left

38. Does your child breathe through their mouth?

( ) Yes, all day.

( ) Yes, but only at night.

( ) Yes, but sometimes he also breathes through his nose.

( ) No, he only breathes through his nose.

( ) I don't know.

39. *Has* the child *ever* breathed through its mouth?

( ) Yes___________________________ . Up to what age?   What is the reason?

( ) No, he has never breathed through his mouth.

( ) I don't know.

40. Does the child sleep with his mouth open?

( ) Yes ( ) No

41. Does your child snore?

( ) Yes   ( ) No

42. Is your child a restless sleeper?

( ) Yes   ( ) No

43. Does your child have frequent colds or flu?

( ) Yes. How many times a year? ____________________

( ) No

44. Does your child have allergic rhinitis?

( ) Yes

( ) No

( ) I don't know what that is.

45. Has your child often had tonsillitis?

( ) Yes

( ) No

( ) I don't know what that is.

46. Has your child had their tonsils removed?

( ) Yes

( ) No

( ) I don't know what that is.

47. Does your child have adenoids?

( ) Yes

( ) No

( ) *Already had it,* but underwent surgery.

( ) I don't know what that is.

48. *Have* you taken the child to an ENT doctor? ( ) Yes. Why?

( ) No

49. Does your child have bronchitis or asthma?

( ) Yes

( ) No

( ) I don't know.

50. Does your child have a headache?

( ) No

( ) When getting up

( ) At night

( ) During meals

( ) During the day

51. Does your child grind their teeth?

( ) No

( ) Only at night

( ) Only during the day

THE ENTIRE ORTHODONTICS TEAM AT UNIVERSIDADE CIDADE DE SAO PAULO THANKS YOU FOR YOUR VALUABLE COLLABORATION!

APPENDIX B

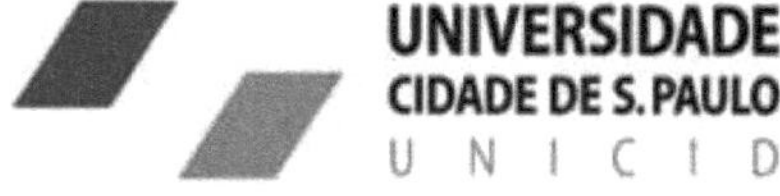

Dentistry course

Discipline of Orthodontics

dental and orthodontic clinical examination form

Date:_______________ ___/___/Examiner: ___________________________________

Course: ( ) Undergraduate   ( ) Master

School: EMEI ____

Student's name: ____

Sex: ( ) M ( )   FI Age: _________

Skin color: ( ) white ( ) black ( ) yellow (oriental) ( ) brown (morena)

1. ODONTOGRAM ▶ Instructions:

II ≡≡If there are decay lesions that compromise occlusion and/or the mesio-distal crown width, draw a rectangle on the corresponding tooth(s);

X Mark the missing deciduous tooth(s) with an "X";

* Are there any fully or partially erupted permanent tooth(s)?

( ) Yes. Which one(s)? ______________________________

( )No

2. *OVERJET*

        ( ) Anterior crossbite (negative passthrough) = -   mm

        ( ) Nil

        ( ) Normal=   + 1 to 2mm

        ( ) Enlarged (gap greater than 2mm) = + _________ mm

        3.   *OVERBITE*

        ( ) Anterior open bite=   - _________mm

( ) Nil

( ) Normal (the upper incisor covers 1/3 of the lower incisor)

( ) Moderately enlarged (upper incisor covers 1/3 to 1/2)

( ) Sharply enlarged (upper incisor covers more than 1/2)

4. RELATIONSHIP OF THE SECOND MOLAR DECADES

Instructions:

During the assessment, consider the side of the arch and the position of at least 1/2 the width of the disto-vestibular cusp of the upper second molar.

Straight terminal plane:

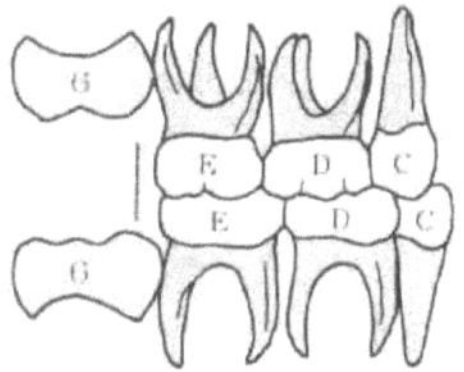

( ) right ( ) left

Mesial step:

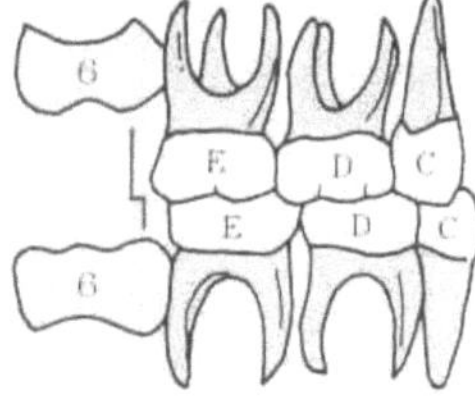

( ) right ( ) left

Distal step:

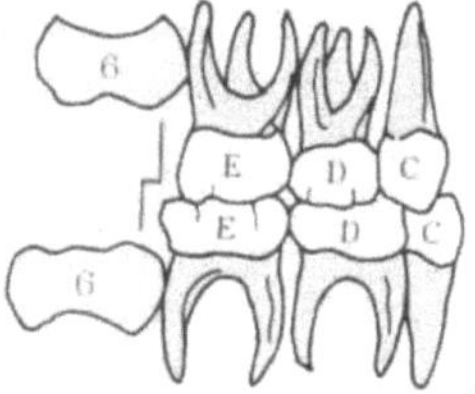

( ) right ( ) left

5. RELATIONSHIP OF DECIDUOUS CANINES

Class 1

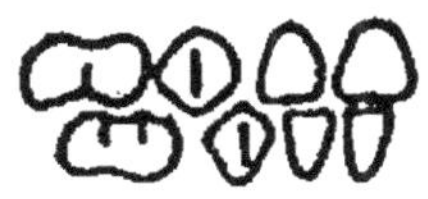

( ) right ( ) left

Class 2

( ) right ( ) left

Class 3

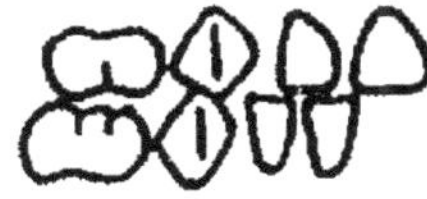

( ) right ( ) left

Top to bottom:

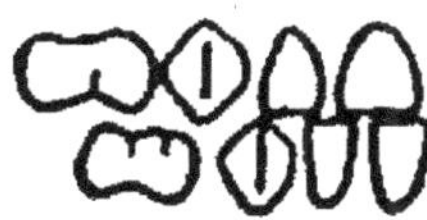

( ) right ( ) left

6. MIDDLE LINE (upper arch/lower arch)

( ) Centralized   ( ) Diverted

7. POSTERIOR CROSSBITE

( ) Absent

( ) Bilateral

( ) Unilateral true: ( ) right ( ) left

( ) Unilateral with functional deviation of the mandible: ( ) right ( ) left

8. DIASTEMAS   ( ) Absent

In the upper arch: ( ) Only primate spaces

                                       ( ) Generalized

In the lower arch: ( ) Absent

                                       ( ) Only primate spaces

                                       ( ) Generalized

9. CROWDING IN THE ANTERIOR REGION

( ) In the upper arch

( ) In the lower arch

( ) non-existent

10. LABiAL SEALING IN REPoUSo

( ) Normal

( ) Present, but with contraction of the peribuccal and mentonian muscles.

( ) Disabled

11. MANDIBULAR MOVEMENT

( ) Symmetrical opening

(   ) Opening with deviation ^ *o the opening begins with the mandible moving and ends with the mandible returning to the midline*

( ) Opening with deflection ^ *the jaw is displaced during the entire opening movement*

12. presence of stallion

( ) No

( ) Yes   ( ) right   ( ) left

13. TOOTH WEAR

( ) incisors

( ) Canines

( ) Molars

( ) Absent

14. INFRA-OCCLUSION OF DECIDUOUS MOLAR

( ) Yes. Which one(s)? _______________________________

( ) No

APPENDIX C

Table 1 - Prevalence of anterior interdental spacing characteristics in the upper arch in Japanese-Brazilians, by age group.

Upper arch

Features	2 to 3 years		4 years		5 to 6 years		Total	
	n	%	n	%	n	%	n	%
absent	34	25,2	26	21,3	28	18,9	88	21,7
primate spaces	36	26,7	37	30,3	41	27,7	114	28,2
generalized	58	43,0	56	45,9	73	49,3	187	46,2
crowding	7	5,2	3	2,5	6	4,1	16	4,0
Total	135	100,0	122	100,0	148	100,0	405	100,0

Table 2 - Frequency comparisons of anterior spacing characteristics between age groups in the upper arch for Japanese-Brazilians.

Upper arch

Comparisons	λ^2	p-value
2-3 versus 4	2.063	0.559
2-3 versus 5-6	2.107	0.550
4 versus 5-6	1.025	0.795

Table 3 - Prevalence of anterior interdental spacing characteristics in the lower arch in Japanese-Brazilians, by age group.

Lower arch

Features	2 to 3 years		4 years		5 to 6 years		Total	
	n	%	n	%	n	%	n	%
absent	34	25,2	36	29,5	37	25,0	107	26,4
primate spaces	21	15,6	19	15,6	22	14,9	62	15,3
generalized	72	53,3	62	50,8	82	55,4	216	53,3
crowding	8	5,9	5	4,1	7	4,7	20	4,9
Total	135	100,0	122	100,0	148	100,0	405	100,0

Table 4 - Frequency comparisons of anterior spacing characteristics between age groups in the lower arch for Japanese-Brazilians.

Lower arch

Comparisons	λ^2	p-value
2-3 versus 4	0.941	0.816
2-3 versus 5-6	0.269	0.966

4 versus 5-6	0.849	0.838

Table 5 - Prevalence of anterior interdental spacing characteristics in the upper arch in Yucoderms, by age group.

Upper arch

Features	2 to 3 years		4 years		5 to 6 years		Total	
	n	%	n	%	n	%	n	%
absent	14	23,0	40	22,4	63	23,3	117	22,9
primate spaces	18	29,5	39	21,8	60	22,2	117	22,9
generalized	25	41,0	95	53,1	136	50,4	256	50,2
crowding	4	6,6	5	2,8	11	4,1	20	3,9
Total	61	100,0	179	100,0	270	100,0	510	100,0

Table 6 - Frequency comparisons of anterior spacing characteristics between age groups in the upper arch for leucodermas.

Upper arch

Comparisons	λ^2	p-value
2-3 versus 4	4.198	0.241
2-3 versus 5-6	2.703	0.440
4 versus 5-6	0.703	0.872

Table 7 - Prevalence of anterior interdental spacing characteristics in the lower arch in leucoderms, by age group.

Lower arch

Features	2 to 3 years		4 years		5 to 6 years		Total	
	n	%	n	%	n	%	n	%
absent	17	27,9	37	20,7	65	24,1	119	23,3
primate spaces	7	11,5	20	11,2	37	13,7	64	12,6
generalized	29	47,5	105	58,7	128	47,4	262	51,4
crowding	8	13,1	17	9,5	40	14,8	65	12,8

	61	100,0	179	100,0	270	100,0	510	100,0
Total	61	100,0	179	100,0	270	100,0	510	100,0

Table 8 - Frequency comparisons of anterior spacing characteristics between age groups in the lower arch for leucodermas.

Lower arch

Comparisons	Z^2	p-value
2-3 versus 4	2.630	0.452
2-3 versus 5-6	0.575	0.902
4 versus 5-6	6.116	0.106

APPENDIX D

Table 1 - Results of the Chi-Square test using the Bonferroni correction for multiple comparisons.

Japanese-Brazilians - Lower Arc

	Comparisons			
	Male		Female	
Features	3-4 years X 5-6 years		3-4 years X 5-6 years	
	X^2	p-value	X2	p-value
primate spaces	0,424	0,515	0,277	0,599
generalized spaces	0,054	0,817	0,668	0,414
crowding	1,735	0,188	2,067	0,150
lack of spaces	0,143	0,706	0,367	0,545

*The total significance level adopted was 5%, the differences in each individual test were considered statistically significant when p-value <0.00625.

Table 2 - Results of the Chi-Square test using the Bonferroni correction for multiple comparisons.

Japanese-Brazilians - Lower Arc

	Comparisons			
	3-4 years		5-6 years	
Features	Male X Female		Male X Female	
	X^2	p-value	X2	p-value
primate spaces	1,351	0,245	0,029	0,865
generalized spaces	1,286	0,257	0,134	0,714
crowding	1,346	0,246	2,503	0,114

| lack of spaces | 2,715 | 0,099 | 1,115 | 0,291 |

*The total significance level adopted was 5%, the differences in each individual test were considered statistically significant when the p-value was <0.00625.

Table 3 - Results of the Chi-Square test using the Bonferroni correction for multiple comparisons.

Japanese-Brazilians - Upper Arc

Features	Comparisons			
	Male		Female	
	3-4 years X 5-6 years		3-4 years X 5-6 years	
	X2	p-value	X2	p-value
primate spaces	0,360	0,549	0,129	0,720
generalized spaces	0,009	0,925	1,449	0,229
crowding	1,374	0,241	0,974	0,324
lack of spaces	0,000	0,990	1,944	0,163

*The total significance level adopted was 5%, the differences in each individual test were considered statistically significant when p-value <0.00625.

Table 4 - Results of the Chi-Square test using the Bonferroni correction for multiple comparisons.

Japanese-Brazilians - Upper Arc

Features	Comparisons			
	3-4 years		5-6 years	
	Male X Female		Male X Female	
	X^2	p-value	X2	p-value
primate spaces	0,177	0,674	0,291	0,589
generalized spaces	0,114	0,735	0,476	0,490
crowding	0,831	0,362	1,486	0,223
lack of spaces	0,184	0,668	0,780	0,377

*The total significance level adopted was 5%, the differences in each individual test were considered statistically significant when p-value <0.00625.

Table 5 - Results of the Chi-Square test using the Bonferroni correction for multiple comparisons.

Leucodermas - Lower arch

| Features | Comparisons | |
	Male	Female

	3-4 years X 5-6 years		3-4 years X 5-6 years	
	X2	p-value	X2	p-value
primate spaces	1,432	0,232	0,000	0,992
generalized spaces	0,138	0,710	5,170	0,023
crowding	0,253	0,615	6,050	0,014
lack of spaces	0,018	0,894	0,478	0,490

*The total significance level adopted was 5%, the differences in each individual test were considered statistically significant when p-value <0.00625.

Table 6 - Results of the Chi-Square test using the Bonferroni correction for multiple comparisons.

Leucodermas - Lower Arc

eatures-	Comparisons			
	F 3-4 years		5-6 years	
	Male X Female		Male X Female	
	X^2	p-value	X2	p-value
primate spaces	0,184	0,668	0,677	0,411
generalized spaces	0,211	0,646	2,034	0,154
crowding	1,521	0,217	3,073	0,080
lack of spaces	0,001	0,975	0,758	0,384

*The total significance level adopted was 5%, the differences in each individual test were considered statistically significant when p-value <0.00625.

Table 7 - Results of the Chi-Square test using the Bonferroni correction for multiple comparisons.

Leucodermas - Superior Arch

Features	Comparisons			
	Male		Female	
	3-4 years X 5-6 years		3-4 years X 5-6 years	
	X^2	p-value	X2	p-value
primate spaces	0,196	0,658	0,023	0,880
generalized spaces	0,664	0,415	0,443	0,506
crowding	0,762	0,383	0,915	0,339
lack of spaces	0,026	0,871	0,226	0,634

*The total significance level adopted was 5%, the differences in each individual test were considered statistically significant when the p-value was <0.00625.

Table 8 - Results of the Chi-Square test using the Bonferroni correction for multiple comparisons.

Leucodermas - Superior Arch

Characteristics	Comparisons			
	3-4 years		5-6 years	
	Male X Female		Male X Female	
	X^2	p-value	X2	p-value
primate spaces	0,028	0,867	0,239	0,625
generalized spaces	0,267	0,605	0,961	0,327
crowding	0,195	0,659	1,932	0,164
lack of spaces	0,345	0,557	0,758	0,384

*The total significance level adopted was 5%, the differences in each individual test were considered statistically significant when p-value <0.00625.

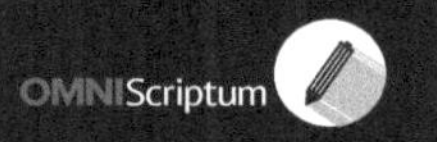

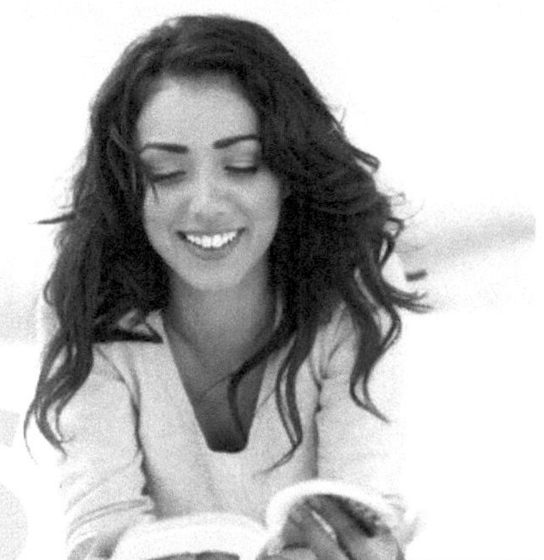

Buy your books fast and straightforward online - at one of world's fastest growing online book stores! Environmentally sound due to Print-on-Demand technologies.

Buy your books online at
www.morebooks.shop

Kaufen Sie Ihre Bücher schnell und unkompliziert online – auf einer der am schnellsten wachsenden Buchhandelsplattformen weltweit! Dank Print-On-Demand umwelt- und ressourcenschonend produzi ert.

Bücher schneller online kaufen
www.morebooks.shop

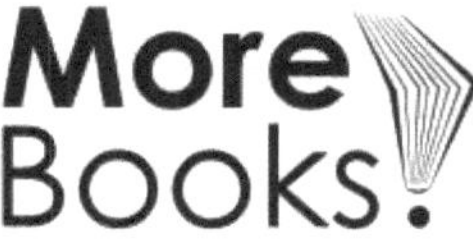

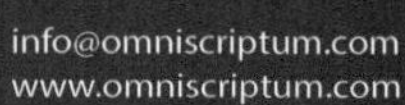